"P

MW01269185

anu

Other Stories of Intensive Care

Medical and Ethical Challenges in the ICU

The following stories were originally published as magazine articles.

"Adult Respiratory Distress" as "A Case for Intensive Care," in *The Gamut*, Fall 1982
"Crusade" as "Hammer Home the Message to Patients Who Smoke," in *Medical Economics*, January 1991
"Pickwickian," in *The Gamut*, Winter 1991
"We Can't Kill Your Mother," in *Medical Economics*, March 1991
"Extraordinary Care" as "Mr. Bowman's Solution," in *The Saturday Evening Post*, April 1991

Published by Lakeside Press
5124 Mayfield Road, # 191
Cleveland, Ohio 44124

For book orders:
1-800-247-6553

Cover Design by Pitt Studios, Cleveland

This book is dedicated to the MICU nurses at my hospital.

Acknowledgement: I would like to thank Dr. Reuben Swimmer for his generous time in reviewing these stories and his encouragement along the way.

Publisher's Cataloging in Publication Information
(Prepared by Quality Books Inc.)

Martin, Lawrence, 1943-
    "Pickwickian" and other stories of intensive care: medical and ethical challenges in the ICU / Lawrence Martin. --
    p. cm.
    Includes bibliographical references and index.
    ISBN 1-879653-04-4

    1. Critical care medicine--Case studies--Popular works. 2. Critical care medicine--Moral and ethical aspects. 3. Medicine--Miscellanea. I. Title

RC96.7   616.028
                                        91-61828
                                        MARC

"PICKWICKIAN"

and Other Stories of Intensive Care

TABLE OF CONTENTS

PREFACE

Did you ever wonder what happens when a patient enters 'Intensive Care'? What goes on behind those doors marked **AUTHORIZED PERSONNEL ONLY**? How do doctors and nurses treat the most complex of medical diseases? And how do they react when patients just don't get better, no matter what modern medicine has to offer? Is the ICU all high tech, impersonal care, or is there a place for the old-fashioned bedside doctor?

You'll find answers to these questions and more in this collection of stories based on real patients cared for in a medical intensive care unit. Like Harold Switek, too ill to leave MICU, too psychotic to stay. And Willie the Yellow Man, whose love affair with alcohol exceeded anything you've ever seen. You'll meet a young socialite hospitalized with rapid onset of total paralysis. Will she ever hug her kids again? And another woman about to have her baby during a terrifying — and life-threatening — asthma attack. Then there's the young accountant who slept in coma — for six months!

You'll join doctors as they care for patients with out-of-control diabetes, severe hypertension, kidney failure and acute psychosis. And you'll come across people you probably wouldn't want to meet anywhere else — like the drug pusher who took one sniff too many of cocaine and the heroin addict with AIDS. Will either patient survive his stay in MICU? And the markedly obese woman whose story gave title to this book. Will she ever lose weight and regain her drive to breathe?

Patients profiled in these stories were hospitalized over the past decade in Memorial Medical Center, a university-affiliated, mid-western teaching hospital. At Memorial the *medical* ICU is separate from the *surgical* intensive care unit, which cares for post-operative patients and trauma victims. MICU is also separate from the *coronary* care unit, where patients are sent with heart attack and other cardiac emergencies.

Whatever the physical arrangement, every sizable hospital handles the same problems and encounters the same ethical dilemmas. Like elderly, senile Mr. Zigson who is trying to die a natural death. Only problem: he has no family. Should the doctors leave him alone or 'do everything'? And the nursing home patient who is awake and alert, but can only live connected to a breathing machine. The patient says she wants to die and her daughter demands that the ventilator be disconnected so "mother can die." Can doctors honor such a request? Can they *ignore* it?

The first chapter ("Rounds") gives an overview of intensive care rounds and how the MICU operates. Succeeding chapters are each devoted to one or two patients and the challenges they present. To preserve patient anonymity all names have been changed as well as some of the descriptive detail.

Medical jargon is kept to a necessary minimum and most unfamiliar terms are described or defined when introduced; a Glossary is also provided at the end of the book. Because many diseases and clinical situations are covered I've also indexed the book so you can readily look up any particular area of interest.

Finally, I've included a short bibliography of works in a similar genre as *"Pickwickian" and other Stories of Intensive Care.* I am not the first, and will certainly not be the last, medical professional to write about his or her patients, and some listing of other works is called for. In a literary sense doctors and nurses are privileged; what we see in our daily jobs is more than enough to fill many interesting books. We just have to find the time and inclination to tell others about what we do, and to make the work seem as interesting in print as it is in real life.

Lawrence Martin, M.D.

1. ROUNDS

I greeted the two new interns. "Welcome to MICU. I'm Dr. Martin. I run the unit and will be rounding with you this month. How does it feel to be starting your internship?"

"Scary," said Deborah Hafly, a petite and energetic woman who came to Memorial with top recommendations. She and her partner on this rotation, Michael Highland, were both excellent students and promised to be good interns.

It was July 1, the beginning of another academic year at Memorial Medical Center. As Director of Memorial's medical intensive care unit, it's my job to supervise and teach house staff and help manage patients admitted to our 8-bed ward.

"You've met the medical resident Jerry Clark, and been assigned your patients?"

"Yes," said Deborah. "He assigned us our patients this morning. We each have four."

"Good. Well, let's make rounds."

MICU occupies a large rectangular space on the second floor of the hospital. The 'unit,' as it is often referred to, consists of eight single-bed rooms arranged in a broad-based 'U' shape, in the center of which is the nursing station. On either side of the nursing station double doors lead to the hallway and family waiting area.

All the patient rooms are fronted by sliding glass doors that can be 'broken' open for quick access; drapes across the doors provide privacy when necessary. Each patient can be 'wired' so that his or her cardiac rhythm is continuously displayed on monitors at the nursing station.

The nurse-patient ratio in MICU is as high as one-to-one when every patient is critically ill. Despite the appellation 'intensive,' however, not all MICU patients are critical. On average, when the unit is full, five nurses per shift can provide excellent care. On the regular hospital wards, which occupy floors five through 12 at Memorial, the average ratio is one registered nurse per eight patients.

MICU rounds are open to anyone on the staff who may have something to contribute. Besides myself (or another staff physician) rounds include two interns, the supervising resident, one or more nurses, and a respiratory therapist. Also participating, on occasion, are medical and nursing students, various consultants and private attending physicians, and a social worker.

If Memorial was not a teaching hospital my job would be much more difficult, perhaps impossible. Most MICU patients require constant management, something not easily done over the phone, or even during brief hospital visits. Physicians must always be available to order medications, adjust ventilator settings, put in catheters, talk to families, examine and treat new admissions, and transfer patients to the regular wards. Private, office-based physicians who send their patients to MICU are thankful for the housestaff and round-the-clock physician coverage. Without interns and residents we could not provide the excellent care Memorial's MICU is known for.

Housestaff, although licensed MDs, are in training and not certified in any specialty. They must be supervised throughout their three or more years of hospital internship and residency. Interns, fresh out of medical school, are supervised by the junior resident, he or she by the senior resident, and all the housestaff by the chief resident, full-time staff and visiting physicians.

Physician training is a dynamic, patient-centered process. Lectures occupy no more than an hour a day. Most of the learning comes from supervised, hands-on patient care, supplemented by reading journals and textbooks.

*   *   *

I took the new interns over to room 1 where we met Dr. Clark and the head nurse.

"Let me introduce you to Marsha Ligner, MICU's head nurse. Marsha, this is Deborah Hafly and Michael Highland, our two new interns."

"Welcome to MICU," she said. "Glad to have you aboard." Turning to me, Marsha continued, "Dr. Martin, who can we transfer out this morning?"

"I don't know. Do we need a bed?"

"Yes. The ER just called. They have an overdose that needs to come up."

I turned to Dr. Clark. "Who can go out?"

"I just put Mr. Jones up for transfer. As soon as a bed's ready he can go."

"OK. Marsha, find us a bed upstairs for Mr. Jones. Tell Patient Placement not to drag their feet. I know there are empty beds on the wards." Marsha nodded. She would make one or two phone calls and Mr. Jones would soon be transferred.

"Is the ER patient intubated?" I asked.

"Not as far as I know," said Dr. Clark.

"OK. Well, let's start rounds. We'll see the new patient as soon as he arrives. Or is it she?"

"A 20-year-old woman. She OD'd on tricyclics."

I stood with my back to the sliding glass doors of Room 1, chart rack and housestaff before me. We were also joined by two of the MICU nurses and a respiratory therapist.

"Has everyone met Dr. Hafly and Dr. Highland?" Everyone had. I addressed the two interns, the only new people on the team. "We round at ten each morning. You should be up to date on your patients by the time rounds begin. Today is an exception of course. Also, we require that you write a chart note on each of your patients every day. You need to list all their medical problems, all drugs they are receiving, and all the tubes entering or exiting their body. Dr. Clark already went over this requirement with you, didn't he?" They nodded yes.

"Good. Jerry, why don't you briefly present each patient as we go around." Jerry Clark, 28, had been the MICU resident in June and was staying another day to orient the new interns. He knew all the patients.

"OK. In room one we have Mr. Hewlett Jones. He's a sixty-seven-year-old gentleman admitted June twenty seventh, with a CVA."

"What's a CVA?" I asked Deborah.

"Cerebrovascular accident," she answered matter-of-factly.

"Jerry, did Mr. Jones have an accident?" I wanted to send a signal early in the month: avoid jargon if possible.

Dr. Clark showed a knowing smile. He had been through this routine with me before. In the spirit of the new year he played it straight — almost.

"No, Dr. Martin," he said, with a trace of sarcasm. "He had a stroke. There was no accident."

"I see. Then why do you call it a 'cerebrovascular *accident?'* Why didn't you — why don't we — just say Mr. Jones had a stroke and be done with it?"

The interns stared in mild disbelief. What kind of rounds were these? English 101? Every new MD has heard the term 'CVA' a hundred times, always meaning a stroke of some sort. Drs. Hafly and Highland had never before heard anyone question the term.

"I don't know," admitted Dr. Clark. "That's just what everyone calls it. I know it makes no sense."

"I agree. It's just one of those terms that gets introduced into medicine, and no one ever questions. OK, go on."

"Well, he had a stroke, a spontaneously-occurring blood clot that blocked his left middle cerebral artery. The clot paralyzed his right side and left him aphasic, but I think he's getting better. Neurology's following him and he's ready for transfer."

We went in to Mr. Jones's room to say good by. Reflecting the crossover of nerve pathways, the right side of his body was limp from a blockage in the left side of his brain. Since the speech center is on the left Mr. Jones couldn't talk, but he recognized us and understood conversation. I explained that he was being transferred out of MICU, that he was improving and with continued physical therapy had an excellent prognosis for recovery. He understood. We left Mr. Jones and rolled the chart rack over to Room 2, stopping in front of the closed glass doors.

"This is Mr. Boykin," said Dr. Clark. "He's a thirty-four-year-old man admitted June twenty ninth with a severe asthma attack. He's improved but we want to continue IV steroids and inhaled bronchodilators another day. His peak flow is up to one forty."

Through the glass we saw a young man in mild respiratory distress, a state made apparent by a fast breathing rate.

"Who's got Mr. Boykin?"

"Deborah."

"OK. Deborah, did you learn about peak flow at your medical school?"

"I didn't have that much experience managing asthma patients. I think I only had one asthmatic on my medicine clerkship."

"Well, you'll become an expert here. Peak flow is the best single breathing test to follow the progress of an asthmatic. It takes only a few seconds and if done properly the test is fairly reproducible."

I asked Greg, our respiratory therapist, to get the peak flow meter so I could demonstrate the test. He went into Mr. Boykin's room and brought back a round, metal instrument the size of a small kitchen clock. A handle on the side of the peak flow meter allows the patient to hold the instrument horizontal while blowing into a mouthpiece situated above the handle. A long needle on the face of the meter deflects when air is blown into the mouthpiece; the harder the blow the greater the deflection. A slight 'puff' into the mouthpiece by a normal adult will register at least 150 liters/minute peak flow. A maximal effort will register at least 400 liters/minute.

I inserted a cardboard mouthpiece into the meter and handed it to Deborah. "Deborah, just put your lips around the mouthpiece and give a little puff." She did as instructed and the needle deflected to 180.

"Now reset the needle and take a deep breath, then blow out with all your strength." The needle went to 495.

"OK. Now let's go see Mr. Boykin." He sat in bed, a strong, virile patient humbled by his asthma.

"How do you feel? Are you any better since you've come in?"

"Oh, much better," he said, with conviction. But how much better? You can be fooled by patients. A 30% improvement from a severe asthma attack can make the patient feel like a million bucks, at least at rest. He was still breathing faster than normal and I heard wheezing on exam.

I inserted a fresh mouthpiece and asked Mr. Boykin to do the peak flow maneuver. He took in a deep breath and blew as hard as he could: 170. I asked him to repeat the effort. The needle went to 168.

"Well, you still have a way to go. Your peak flow is still

reduced. We're going to keep you here today and continue the intravenous medication. You might be able to go upstairs tomorrow." I thanked him and we stepped outside.

"What do you think?" I asked the interns.

"I'm surprised," said Dr. Highland. He doesn't look that short of breath."

"I agree. I think he may have chronic asthma. The only way to gauge severity of asthma is with the peak flow or some similar measurement. Despite maximal effort he couldn't get above 170 on the peak flow." I looked at Deborah. "You did better than that with almost no effort. He looks strong but if he ran a race with you right now it would be no contest."

"What's going to happen to him?" asked Deborah.

"Too soon to tell," I said. He's much better than yesterday, that's for sure. If he can't reach a higher peak flow despite several more days of IV therapy, then his impairment is chronic. He used to smoke heavily so that may be contributing. Anyway, it's too early to say. We'll watch him in MICU one more day, then send him upstairs if he remains stable."

We moved to room 3. "This is Mr. Denton Smith," said Dr. Clark. "He came in last night with a gastrointestinal hemorrhage. He's a heavy alcoholic. GI's already 'scoped him."

"What'd they find?" The gastroenterology service is good at putting 'scopes,' long flexible tubes with a light on the end and a channel through the middle, into the stomach of bleeding patients.

"A large duodenal ulcer. Here's a picture."

Dr. Clark opened up the chart. Taped in the middle of a progress note was an amazingly sharp, digitized photo of an intestinal ulcer. In the middle of a normal stomach lining sat a white dime-sized patch, and in the middle of that a tiny dab of red. I read the handwritten legend under the photo. "Eroding gastric ulcer with bleeding vessel as shown. Vessel cauterized."

"Has his bleeding stopped?"

"Yes, but GI wants us to observe him for another day. We've given him a total of three units of blood."

"OK. I see in the note that he has continued to drink. Was he drunk when he came in?"

"No, he says he hasn't had anything to drink in three days. So we're also going to watch for DT's [delirium tremens]."

"Didn't anyone ever tell him to quit drinking?" I asked. It was a rhetorical question. "What's his hematocrit?"

"It was 23% on admission. After the three units it's up to 30."

Suddenly two nurses from the station began running toward room 7. The first to arrive punched open the door and the other one hauled in the red crash cart. We arrived seconds later. The patient was Mrs. Waldstein, a 76-year-old woman with end-stage kidney and heart disease. The day before she had received a shunt in her right arm for kidney dialysis. We had spent considerable time with her and her family discussing such issues as quality of life, what she could expect with dialysis, possible therapy without it, and so on. In the end she said she wasn't ready to die or become a vegetable, and accepted dialysis.

Even so, her kidney doctor was concerned about whether her heart was strong enough to withstand three times a week dialysis. She had suffered two heart attacks in the past year. Two days earlier she was admitted to MICU with pulmonary edema — excess fluid in the lungs from kidney and heart failure. Now her heart had suddenly stopped beating altogether. If we did nothing in the next two minutes she would be dead.

"Ambu bag!"

"Epinephrine!"

"Call anesthesiology!"

"They're called."

"Let's get a rhythm strip."

Dr. Clark positioned himself at the head of the bed and began ventilating her with an Ambu bag while I took up chest compressions. One of the nurses began infusing epinephrine into an arm vein while another stuck Mrs. Waldstein's femoral artery for a blood gas sample.

"Any heart beat?"

"Stop pumping for a second." My pumping was creating an artificial heart beat which could mask the patient's own.

"I'll give you three seconds," I said. "Anything more and she's lost."

"Still flat line."

"Give an amp of calcium." The nurse handling drugs infused the calcium.

"Give an amp of bicarbonate. She's acidotic from her renal failure. Somebody please listen to her chest." Deborah complied.

"Good breath sounds when you're bagging," Dr. Martin, we've got a rhythm. Look's idioventricular."

"Any pulse?"

"Only when you pump. Can you stop for a minute?"

"Impossible. A minute is eternity." I stopped for four seconds.

"I feel something. Let me check her blood pressure."

The anesthesiologist arrived. Good, I thought, it's Josh; he's one of the best. Anesthesiologists are expert at intubating patients, so we always call them for a cardiopulmonary arrest. By now there were at least seven people in the room.

Josh went to the head of her bed.

"Hold off intubating for a second, Josh," I said. "Let me see what her rhythm is."

"If she's got a pressure you still want her intubated?" he asked.

"Yes. I want to make sure she's adequately oxygenated and ventilated. This can happen again. What's her blood pressure?"

"I'm getting 90 by palpation," said one of the nurses. Do you still want epi to run in?"

"Yes. Now, let's get her intubated."

Josh expertly slipped the foot-long tube into Mrs. Waldstein's throat while I held my pumping. Seconds later I resumed chest compressions. Dr. Clark continued bagging her, only now he was pumping fresh air through the endotracheal tube, a direct conduit into her lungs.

"Looks like a nodal rhythm, Dr. Martin."

"Good. I'll stop pumping." I felt for a pulse in her groin and felt a repetitive thump against my finger tips. "Look's like she's gonna make it. Let's get a ventilator hooked up and also another blood gas. Stop the epinephrine."

We stayed in Mrs. Waldstein's room another twenty minutes, to make sure she was stable. The nurses' initial response to the cardiac arrest was so quick I doubted she had suffered any brain damage.

*   *   *

On leaving Mrs. Waldstein's room I noted that Deborah and Michael were staring rather idly at the cardiac monitor, Michael with hands in his pockets. They felt insecure in the midst of this emergency and sought to reassure them.

"Don't worry. By the end of the month you'll know exactly what to do. I promise." Affecting nonchalance I added, "Let's resume rounds." We moved on to room 4.

"This is John Popola," said Dr. Clark. "He's seventy-two, with end-stage Alzheimer's. He was sent here for pneumonia and respiratory failure. His sputum culture's growing *pseudomonas aeruginosa*. We have him on gentamicin and piperacillin. We can't get him off the ventilator until his pneumonia clears. He's DNR." Before us was a man looking perhaps ten years older, white hair, face grizzly, eyes sunken in. He was not awake, an effect of sedation given to relieve respiratory distress.

"You two know what DNR means, I assume."

"Do not resuscitate," said Deborah.

"Right. So why's he connected to the ventilator?" I asked. No answer.

"Jerry, if he's 'Do Not Resuscitate,' why the ventilator? Isn't that resuscitation?"

"He wasn't DNR until after he was intubated. Then the family decided they didn't want any more heroics. They don't want him resuscitated again if his heart stops or he crashes. So we made him DNR."

"What family?"

"His wife is deceased. We talked to a sister and his son. They both agreed."

"Michael, how does being DNR affect the care of a ventilator patient?" This was not a fair question for the first day of internship, but I wanted the interns to think about it anyway.

"I don't know," he said.

"It just means we don't add more life support," I explained. "Otherwise it doesn't affect the care at all. We'll treat Mr. Popola's pneumonia in the usual way, and will do our best to get him safely off the ventilator. In some circumstances no treatment may be given a DNR patient, but that's not the case with Mr. Popola."

"Does the family have to sign for DNR status at Memorial?" Michael asked.

"No. You just have to write a note in the chart documenting that you talked to the patient if he's competent, or to the family if the patient is not."

We reviewed the ventilator settings and blood gases, then all of Mr. Popola's medications. There was still a way to go before he could breathe unassisted by the machine. We moved on.

"In room five we have Elsie McKnight," Dr. Clark said. "She's a tylenol overdose."

"Looks like a young woman to me," I said. At that, Dr. Clark rolled his eyes and made a here-we-go-again face. I ignored him.

"Suppose a patient pointed to you and said, 'There's a stethoscope,' or 'here we have a reflex hammer.' "

"OK, OK," Dr. Clark said, in a manner of 'enough, enough.' Actually he took my comments good-naturedly. They were really intended to impress the interns and, perhaps, change in some minuscule way the language of medicine. Doctors already well into their post-graduate training, like Dr. Clark, were usually beyond my message.

"Miss McKnight is a twenty-five-year-old woman who *took* an overdose of Tylenol tablets. When she came to the ER they measured her acetaminophen [tylenol] level; it was twenty-four."

"Michael, do you have any question about that? What would you want to know at that point?"

"Was she breathing?"

"No, I don't mean about her vital signs. Obviously you want to know if a patient is breathing, if her heart is beating, and so forth. I mean, given that she took tylenol and you have a blood level of the drug, what specific question should you ask?"

Jerry thought for a moment. "What else did she take?"

"Well, that's important too, but let's assume it's only tylenol. It is, as far as we know, isn't it Jerry?" Jerry nodded yes.

"OK, it's only tylenol. What specific question do you need to ask?"

"I'm not sure what you're getting at, Dr. Martin."

I turned to the other intern. "Deborah?"

"When did she take the pills?"

"EXACTLY. You need to know *when* she took the pills because treatment depends on that information *and* the blood level. What's the story, Jerry?"

"The blood tylenol level was drawn about six hours after she took the pills."

"OK. What would you do?" I addressed both interns. Deborah spoke up first.

"At that level I would definitely give acetylcystein."

"Right. We gave it to her," I said. "Otherwise, what can happen?"

"Severe liver toxicity."

"Right." Clearly, of the two new interns Deborah was sharper.

* * *

We went in to see Ms. McKnight. Not the most pleasant person, she so far had refused to talk to anyone. A tall, thin, flat-chested young woman, she sat up in bed with arms crossed and glared straight ahead. Based on a suicide note and the number of pills she took, her attempt was no gesture. She was angry because we saved her life.

"How do you feel?" I asked. She looked at me, then away, and did not answer. Her monitor showed normal vital signs. By now her risk for liver toxicity was minimal because of the acetylcystein treatment, a drug which prevents tylenol from forming a toxic metabolite. As soon as she could be evaluated by psychiatry she would be transferred from MICU. I saw no point in spending more time in her room. We moved on to room 6.

"Here we have the strangest case of all. Everyone meet 'Jane Doe,' " said Dr. Clark.

"That's not her real name, is it?" asked Deborah.

"No. They found her in a parking lot. Comatose, no identification. She's been here since yesterday morning. I'm told she was intubated in front of a Cadillac. Anyway she has severe aspiration pneumonia and is on the ventilator with one hundred percent oxygen. Right now, except for Mrs. Waldstein, she's our sickest patient. She's got a chance to make it. Nothing here that's irreversible."

"Jerry, did you call the police?"

"Yes, I called and asked if there is a missing persons report on someone of her description. A black woman about sixty years old. They haven't got back to me yet."

As we talked the interns took notes. They seemed overwhelmed, but in less than two days they would know everyone in detail, including any new arrivals.

We stopped in room 7 to see Mrs. Waldstein again. Her cardiac rhythm and blood pressure were holding steady. Arterial blood gases were adequate, albeit with artificial ventilation. She seemed in no immediate danger so we moved on to room 8.

"Last but not least, room eight, Marie Jackson. Very sad case," said Dr. Clark. Before us lay an 80-year-old woman completely comatose and connected to a ventilator.

Jerry opened her chart and pointed to the top of one page. "What do you see there?" he asked the interns.

"A date."

"What's the date?"

"May third."

"Two months. She came to Memorial on May third for a dementia workup. Her private [physician] ordered all the right tests, but nobody ever asked her or her family about what to do if she needed resuscitation. Well, she went for a CAT scan of her brain and guess what happened?"

"She arrested?"

"Right on the table. It was a mess, trying to get her intubated. To make a long story short she must have been apneic for a good five to ten minutes. After her cardiac arrest, which was on May sixth, she developed every complication. Pneumonia, kidney failure, sepsis. We've treated everything. Family won't let go. Neurology agrees she has severe hypoxic encephalopathy, with almost zero chance for meaningful recovery. Actually they said that on June 1. Here we are a month later."

Ms. Jackson — tube in throat, life supported by machine — had her eyes open but demonstrated no awareness of us or of her surroundings. She just stared past us. Periodically there was a twitching, writhing movement of her face and mouth, an indication of partially suppressed seizure activity.

"Why does she need a ventilator?" asked Deborah.

"Good question," I said. "Hypoxic brain damage by itself doesn't usually require artificial ventilation. Unfortunately, her pneumonia was so severe that her lungs became permanently damaged. She probably has also some emphysema, from years of smoking. Anyway we can't get her off the machine.

"What happens when you try to wean her?" Deborah asked.

"We tried once. She lasted a day and then developed respiratory distress. The family was given the option of not connecting her back to the ventilator but they couldn't agree. Some relatives said yes, some said no. Finally guilt prevailed and they asked us to reconnect her. For that reason we are not even trying to wean her from the ventilator. She would probably arrest again and it would be a bad scene."

"There's also the problem that it happened in the hospital," Dr. Clark added.

"Yes," I said. "But the family's not talking lawsuit or anything. It's just that because it happened here everyone is skittish about pushing them to let her go. I'd love to get Mrs. Jackson out of MICU but the ward isn't ready for her just yet."

The interns just shook their heads. It would take time to adjust to this reality of modern medicine: with all our machines we sometimes do more harm than good.

"Well, let's go look at x-rays. Afterwards you can come back and get to know your patients in more detail." We went to the x-ray viewing room across the hall from MICU. About ten minutes later the phone rang in the viewing room. One of the house officers answered the phone and took a message from MICU, then relayed the information to the rest of us.

"The overdose is here."

Comment

In these stories dialogue is presented pretty much as it is spoken on rounds. You are right to be offended if you ever hear patients referred to as a diagnosis or organ; phrases like "this overdose," "that gallbladder," and "the heart" are abhorent when they substitute for "Mr. Jones" or "Mrs. Wilson." Unfortunately, doctors and nurses are incorrigible users of jargon and it is not an easy habit to break. I apologize for any conversation that may offend the reader. Despite the way some doctors and nurses may on occasion communicate with one another, in my experience they invariably speak to patients and families in a manner that is most respectful.

2. OVERDOSE

Judy Bilowitz was only 20 when she came to MICU but this was not her first hospital admission. She was diagnosed as a "depressed personality" shortly after puberty and as a teenager spent two long periods in Weathergill Pavilion, the state's top psychiatric hospital. Judy came from a prosperous family and could afford the best care.

With the aid of expensive tutoring Judy made it through a private girls' prep school, graduating at 19. Unlike most everyone else in her class she did not go to college or take time off for travel. Instead she stayed home with her parents and 15-year-old brother, an outgoing and mentally healthy sophomore.

Judy's father owned a scrap metal company and her mother was on the board of several important charities. The parents' financial and social success only heightened the pain of Judy's illness; their older child simply held no promise. She had no interest in college and was too withdrawn to find and keep a job.

Judy also had little interest in boys, nor they in her. Though attractive physically — she possessed a slim, well-proportioned body, fair complexion and features that made for a pretty face, with straight brown hair — her inattention and blunted affect tended to repel the opposite sex. Boys unaware of her psychiatric illness usually considered her 'screwed up,' or 'weird.'

She was not a virgin. At 15 she became pregnant and had an abortion in her eighth week. She was in Weathergill at the time of conception and the offender was thought to be another patient. Tightened supervision during her second hospital stay, at age 17, prevented another sexual liaison. As far as her parents knew Judy used no birth control.

To the outside world Judy at 20 didn't seem to care much about anything. She was incapable of relating to others and had few identifiable interests. Despite every material advantage there was little to occupy her time. She stared at TV much of the day, sometimes read or pretended to read (all her books had pictures), and occasionally worked in the garden.

She had been under the care of three psychiatrists since puberty. Her current therapist was Dr. Erasmus Cohen, a medical school faculty member in his late 30s and, at the time of Judy's MICU admission, considered the ablest psychiatrist on Memorial's staff.

Dr. Cohen's assessment was that Judy suffered from 'schizo-affective disorder associated with depression,' a form of psychosis usually treated with medication. In Dr. Cohen's best clinical judgment she stood to benefit from Triavil, a combination of the antidepressant *amitriptyline* (also marketed alone as Elavil) and the antianxiety drug *perphenazine*.

Triavil comes in various dosages; the dose Dr. Cohen prescribed for Judy was 2-25, twice a day. Each 2-25 tablet contains 2 milligrams (mg) of perphenazine and 25 mg of Elavil. Judy's prescription began in late March, a little over three months before she ended up in MICU.

Judy faithfully took the Triavil and seemed to improve. She became more talkative, took trips with her parents, and joined a local gardening society. Because of the favorable response Dr. Cohen renewed the drug monthly; her last prescription for 60 tablets was filled June 20.

On July 1 Judy didn't come to breakfast as usual. At about 8:30 the maid went to Judy's room and found her unconscious on the bed, the empty Triavil container beside her. There was no suicide note. From this information it was deduced that she took about 40 of the Triavil tablets.

Judy Bilowitz was Memorial Medical Center's first overdose of the new academic year.

*   *   *

Overdoses can be classified as intentional or accidental. Accidental overdose occurs when too much of a drug is taken by mistake; this occurs mainly among children and the confused elderly.

People who intentionally overdose are usually suicidal, although occasionally an excess of drugs is taken "just to get some sleep," or "to cure my headache." Most of the overdose patients admitted to MICU are, like Judy Bilowitz, intentional and suicidal. Only about half leave behind a suicide note.

Would-be suicides may choose either prescription or over-the-counter drugs. OTC drugs such as aspirin and tylenol are, of course, toxic in large doses and can be lethal. Prescription drugs commonly overdosed, besides Triavil, include Elavil and other single-agent antidepressants, Valium and other anti-anxiety medications, lithium (used in manic states), dilantin (seizures), theophylline (asthma), and Darvon (pain).

Elavil belongs to the group of 'tricyclic antidepressants' (TCAs), so called because of their three-ring chemical configuration. TCAs are indicated for "endogenous" depression, a state unrelated to external events. People depressed over real-life problems such as loss of job or divorce generally do not benefit from taking medication.

The usual Elavil dose for outpatients is 50 to 75 mg a day, although twice this amount can be prescribed in some cases. For inpatients, as much as 300 mg a day can be used.

A combination drug like Triavil is particularly helpful in some psychotic patients. The tricyclic fights the depression while the tranquilizer combats any tendency to agitation.

Tricyclics by themselves are also used for other conditions. Imipramine, the first available TCA, is now widely used for childhood enuresis (bedwetting). Elavil, the most frequently prescribed TCA, is also used for chronic pain syndromes.

It is for endogenous depression, however, that TCAs are most often prescribed and that use of the drug presents the greatest hazard. The hazard exists because depressed patients are often suicidal and TCAs are lethal in large doses. The widespread use and potential toxicity of TCAs, plus the nature of the patients, account for three sobering statistics: an estimated 500,000 Americans overdose on TCAs each year; TCAs are the number one cause of fatal overdose; over 70% of successful TCA suicides are pronounced dead *before* reaching the hospital.

It must be accepted that the risk of suicide exists in any severely depressed patient. If the treatment of choice for depression was bottled water we would no doubt see patients suffering water intoxication. They would be bloated but few, if any, would die. Instead the treatment for many patients is a drug that is potentially lethal in large amounts.

The manufacturer's Product Information Guide to Elavil states:

> High doses may cause temporary confusion, disturbed concentration, or transient visual hallucinations. Overdosage may cause drowsiness; hypothermia; tachycardia and other arrhythmic abnormalities; congestive heart failure; dilated pupils; disorders of ocular motility; convulsions; severe hypotension; stupor; and coma.

*   *   *

Judy Bilowitz arrived at Memorial's emergency room at 8:55 a.m., comatose. While one physician took a history from the parents others intubated her and began artificial ventilation. Her stomach was evacuated with a large bore nasogastric tube and then aspirated to remove any residual pill fragments. Activated charcoal, a drug absorbent, was put down the tube to bind any tablets not yet absorbed into the blood.

The ER physicians placed her suicide attempt between 11 p.m. June 30 and 7 a.m. July 1. Had she swallowed the pills after 7 a.m. she would not likely have been in coma 90 minutes later.

It took the ER doctors about two hours to stabilize Judy and transfer her to MICU. I saw her for the first time as she was wheeled into room 1. My first impression was that she looked like a true suicidal patient: young; comatose; pale skin without makeup; hair all frizzed; face distorted by two tubes, one in the mouth and the other in the nose. From just visual inspection I surmised Judy's overdose was no "gesture."

The clear plastic stomach tube, inserted through her left nostril, was now jet black from the charcoal absorbent. This tube would stay in place at least two days so she could receive additional charcoal every 6 hours. The endotracheal tube stuck out from the left side of her mouth and was secured with white adhesive tape that circled her head; it would remain until she could safely breathe on her own.

The physical exam, which I did with the intern Deborah Hafly, can be summarized as follows:

Body temperature: 97.6 degrees.
Pulse: 116/minute (increased)
Blood pressure: 123/82 (normal)
Respiratory rate: 16 (provided by ventilator)
Head: no bruises or any sign of trauma.
Eyes: closed; no eye makeup; pupils dilated equally and
    reactive to light; retinal exam normal.
Ears: normal.
Neck: no stiffness; carotid pulses equal and strong.
Lungs: normal chest movements each time the ventilator
    pushed in air; normal lung sounds as heard with the
    stethoscope.
Heart: normal, except for fast heart rate of 120 beats per
    minute.
Abdomen: no tenderness or swelling.
Arms and legs: normal; no needle marks or scratches.
Genital area: Bladder catheter (inserted in emergency room)
    draining clear yellow urine.
Nervous system: in deep coma; no response to her name but
    responsive to arm pinching by withdrawing her limb;
    tendon reflexes equal and hyperactive in all extremities.
    Eye reflexes and eye movements appropriate, indicating
    no structural brain damage.

After our exam we checked results of tests obtained in the emergency room. Her EKG showed no arrhythmias but the 'QRS' wave pattern generated by the heart's conduction system showed slight widening, a common finding in TCA overdose. We would watch this closely since further widening could signal impending cardiac arrest.

Her chest x-ray was clear, ruling out pulmonary complications such as aspiration pneumonia and pulmonary edema. An arterial blood gas drawn shortly after intubation showed adequate oxygen and carbon dioxide levels. Other blood tests showed no electrolyte imbalance or disease of the kidneys, liver, or pancreas. Her pregnancy test was negative.

"Well," I said to Dr. Hafly, "she looks stable for now. She'll need an arterial line, which the resident can help you with. We'll need to check her blood gases throughout the night. Our job is to support her ventilation and watch for cardiac or neurologic complications. She took about 40 tablets. That's enough Elavil to kill her."

"What about the other ingredient, the perphenazine?"

"I'm not so worried about that. Perphenazine's probably contributing to her coma but it doesn't have the same lethal cardiac and neurologic effects as the tricyclics, at least not in the dose she ingested. By the way, is there an antidote for Elavil overdose?"

Dr. Hafly thought for a moment. "I don't know. I guess not, or she would have received it by now."

"Right. But if a patient develops life threatening side effects, particularly cardiac, we sometimes use IV physostigmine. It blocks the stimulatory effects of the Elavil."

"Why don't we use it now? Her QRS [EKG wave form] is slightly widened."

"Physostigmine has its own side effects and can be dangerous. Besides, it's not an antidote, just another drug to block Elavil's nastier side effects. The EKG should improve as the drug leaves her body. After you put in the A-line read the review on TCA overdose. A copy's at the nursing station."

I gave her the exact reference and went to the waiting area to meet Judy's parents.

*   *   *

Her parents impressed me as decent, hard working people, upper middle class or perhaps even wealthy but not at all pretentious. Of course no one is pretentious when their child is hospitalized, but I have seen parents whose life style and ostentatious behavior seemed to explain their child's psychopathic behavior. I didn't feel that way about Judy's mother or father.

As a parent myself I felt sorry for them. Sorry that they had such a burden of a daughter, that they were denied the pleasure of watching her grow and mature normally and, far worse, that they might lose her to a fatal overdose. I tried to stay professional and show empathy at the same time.

"Right now she's stable," I said. "She's listed as critical but her blood pressure and heart are holding up and all her vital organs are working except for her breathing. The machine will breathe for her until she comes out of coma."

"What are her chances, Doctor?" The questions came from Judy's mother.

"Well, I can't give a definite percentage but I'd say they're better than 50-50. The fact that she reached the hospital alive is a good sign."

"What do you mean?"

"About 70% of people who overdose on drugs like Triavil die before they reach a hospital. It can be a very dangerous drug in the dose Judy took. On the other hand most of the patients who reach the intensive care unit survive the overdose."

"If she makes it will she be...will she be OK?"

"You mean will she have any major impairment?"

"Yes."

"It's impossible to say now. Her heart and kidneys are not damaged, and there is nothing to suggest brain damage so far. If she doesn't wake up within about forty-eight hours we'll do a brain wave study and some other tests to check for brain damage. Right now we can explain her coma by the overdose, so we just have to wait and see how she does."

Judy's parents looked at each other but said nothing. They had no further questions for the moment so I returned to the Unit.

An hour later Judy seized. The seizure started as a jerking movement of the left arm and within seconds progressed to involve her whole body. Her heart rate jumped to 160/minute and respirations became jerky.

The ventilator cannot properly deliver air when the patient bucks and seizes. The machine lets us know things are awry by sounding off a loud alarm: BZZZZZZZZZZ! Every attempt to push air into Judy's lungs met resistance from her jerking diaphragms. BZZZZZZZZZZZ! BZZZZZZZZZZZ!

Other alarms went off. The heart monitor sounded a repetitive PING! PING! because Judy's heart rate was way too fast. Then the IV infusion pump went BEEP-BEEP-BEEP to signal fluid backing up in the tubing, a result of her spasms.

For about a minute there was cacophony and confusion in room 1. BZZZZZZZZZZZ! PING! PING! BEEP-BEEP-BEEP. BZZZZZZZZZZZ! PING! PING! BEEP-BEEP-BEEP. BZZZZZZZZZZZ! BZZZZZZZZZZZ! Through it all Judy's body jerked and shook in the manner typical of grand mal seizure.

The first things to take care of in any life-threatening situation are ABC: airway, breathing, circulation. I disconnected the ventilator from the endotracheal tube and manually pumped air into her lungs with an AMBU bag. Dr. Hafly listened to her lungs to check the results of my effort.

"I hear good air entry in both lungs."

"Blood pressure's holding at about one twelve over sixty-eight," added a nurse.

"Good. Let's give her ten milligrams of Valium and one milligram of physostigmine," I ordered. "Give the Valium first. We've got to break the seizure." About one minute had passed since the seizure began.

"Valium is in."

Thirty seconds later Judy stopped seizing. Valium works that quickly. The only problem is that Valium is short acting. It doesn't prevent recurrence of seizures so a long-acting drug like Dilantin has to be started.

"Let's load her up with Dilantin. Give her seven hundred milligrams over about thirty minutes." I looked up at the monitor and found that her heart was still beating fast at one sixty. "And give the physostigmine," I added.

With the seizure under control I reconnected the endotracheal tube to the ventilator. Next we checked an arterial blood gas and electrocardiogram. The cardiac conduction complex was still slightly widened but not worse than before, and her heart rate was coming down — 135. Blood pressure and urine output were good and there was no apparent organ damage. Her brain might have suffered damage from the seizure but it was too early to tell, especially with all the Valium on board. With dilantin infusing into her arm vein there was nothing more to do, at least for the moment. I went to write some chart notes.

Thirty minutes later Judy seized again. Her second spasm was not as violent as the first one. We again bagged her manually and gave another 10 mg of intravenous Valium. This time her seizure stopped spontaneously, just as the Valium was injected.

ABC. A and B were secure but now C was a problem. Her blood pressure fell from 118/68 before the seizure to a life-threatening 80/40 and her heart rate was back up to 160. Low blood pressure — hypotension — is an ominous sign in TCA overdose. It often precedes cardiac arrest. This was a critical moment.

"Infuse normal saline, wide open. And give two amps of bicarbonate. Also another milligram of physostigmine."

Saline to expand her intravascular blood volume and raise the blood pressure. Bicarbonate to alkalinize her blood and decrease the amount of active TCA. Physostigmine to lower her fast heart rate. If these maneuvers didn't work the next step would be 'pressors,' drugs that have a direct effect on raising blood pressure. Unfortunately pressors also raise the heart rate and Judy's was already sky high.

It was now 1 p.m. Since arriving to MICU Judy had received, all intravenously:

2 mg physostigmine
1000 mg Dilantin
20 mg Valium
2 ampules of sodium bicarbonate
500 cc saline, with more running in rapidly.

My mind was racing. What else to do? I couldn't think of anything. We continued with manual ventilation. The ventilator might make things worse, perhaps lower her blood pressure by forcing air in too quickly. I kept an eye on the overhead monitor, which gave a continuous readout of heart rate, cardiac rhythm, and blood pressure.

"What about dialysis?" Dr. Hafly asked. "Can it be used to

remove TCAs?"

"No," I explained. "Dialysis does nothing to speed removal of Elavil. The drug is mostly bound to large protein molecules which aren't removed with dialysis. It just doesn't work for tricyclics. If she makes it through this crisis we'll continue pumping her stomach with activated charcoal. Otherwise we just have to wait for her body to metabolize the drug — and try to keep her pressure up."

A nurse cut in. "Pressure's ninety over sixty, Dr. Martin. Heart rate one forty."

"Good. Deborah, please listen to her lungs again. All this fluid can throw her into pulmonary edema."

"Her lungs are still clear."

I looked at the monitor. Blood pressure 100/65. Heart rate 135. I relaxed a little. I wouldn't have to tell Judy's parents the worst news imaginable.

*   *   *

Over the next half hour the threat of cardiac arrest diminished as Judy's pressure and heart rate stabilized. We reconnected the ventilator and checked another arterial blood gas. Oxygen and carbon dioxide levels were adequate, thanks in part to the enriched oxygen provided by the ventilator.

Continued coma and need for artificial ventilation meant she was still critical, that she still needed one-on-one nursing care. Every hour Judy's nurses charted blood pressure, respiratory rate (from the ventilator), pulse and cardiac rhythm, urine output, fluid intake, and the level of her coma. Every 4-6 hours they charted arterial blood gases, body temperature, a cardiac rhythm strip, list of medications delivered, and a detailed clinical assessment.

Besides keeping meticulous records the nurses administered drugs and fluids, turned and cleaned her, and changed her bed sheets at least once every eight hours. Judy's care exemplified one immutable fact: no matter how sophisticated the technology a critically ill patient needs constant *human* attention. Patients like Judy live or die on nursing care. Doctors may direct the show but nurses give the care, and Judy had the best.

*   *   *

Judy remained comatose for 36 hours. The evening of the second day she showed the first signs of waking up. Only then did I feel confident she would survive the overdose. Seizures were under control and her blood pressure was steady at 120/74. Her young heart had withstood a massive tricyclic overdose.

As the coma lifted her brain's respiratory center also recovered. By the morning of July 3 she was breathing entirely on her own, so we removed the endotracheal tube. A few minutes later we removed the still-black nasogastric tube.

With both tubes out Judy was on her way to full physical, if not mental, recovery. Neurologic exam showed no defects and her heart rate was a healthy 86 per minute. Her affect was flat but that didn't concern us; it is the norm for patients awakening after a severe overdose. Because of possible delayed cardiac side effects we planned to watch her in MICU until at least July 5.

July 4 was a hospital holiday. We made rounds as usual but all non-emergency tests and procedures were put on hold until the next day. As if in recognition of the holiday Judy was well behaved. She ate some soup and other liquids and made no demands on the staff. We pulled out the bladder catheter and got her out of bed. Her parents were in and out most of the day, obviously grateful for her survival, also worried about what might come next.

On the morning of July 5, now that Judy was awake and could at least respond verbally, Dr. Cohen re-entered the picture. He visited her bedside for about 15 minutes, then recommended a transfer to the hospital's psychiatry ward after her discharge from MICU. There he would reassess her need for antidepressant medication.

"Is she still suicidal?" I asked, and immediately felt foolish over the question. Given her history when would Judy Bilowitz *not* be suicidal?

"She doesn't want to talk about the overdose right now," Dr. Cohen said. "I spent most of the time talking about other aspects

of her life. She's still pretty numb. I think she'll open up more
on Psychiatry." We agreed she could be transferred the next day.

*   *   *

That afternoon, suddenly and without any threat or warning,
Judy began screaming. I was in MICU at the time. My initial
reaction was that she hurt herself; perhaps she fell out of bed or
hit her head. We rushed to her room. She was in bed, eyes half
closed, screaming a high pitched

AAAAYYYYYYYYYYYYYEEEEEEEEEEEEEE!

It was a wail to wake the dead.
We found no evidence for any injury. I shook her and she
quieted down momentarily. Then she looked at us — at me, two
nurses, and Dr. Hafly standing at the bedside — closed her eyes
and turned away.
"GO AWAAAAAY!" she yelled.
LEAVE ME ALONNNNNNE!"
"Judy, what's the matter?," I asked. "What's wrong?"
"Where's GREGORY?" she asked, in a tone as if to demand
we release someone named Gregory.
"Who's Gregory?" I asked one of the nurses, assuming there
was some history I had missed.
"Beats me," the nurse said. "I don't know."
Dr. Hafly didn't know either.
"Judy," I asked. "Who's Gregory? Is he your brother?"
"AAAAAAAYYYYYYYYYYYYYYYYYYYYYEEEEEEEEEE
EEEEEEEEEE!"
"I don't think Gregory's her brother," said the nurse. "I met
him and his name is Jimmy. Should we give her something, Dr.
Martin?"
"No. Her vital signs are stable. Let's just watch her so she
doesn't hurt herself. I'll call Dr. Cohen."
I put in a call to his office but he was unavailable. I told his
answering service it was important and to have him call back as
soon as possible. Judy was in no physical danger but we could

not keep her in MICU like this. At the least her wailing was disruptive. More important, it was probably a sign that she needed to go back on psychiatric medication.

One of the nurses tried to calm Judy but it was no use. Judy wasn't seeking reassurance or a kind word. She didn't want anything except 'Gregory,' and it wasn't even clear that she wanted him — if Gregory was a him.

Dr. Cohen finally called back about an hour later. I told him what had taken place.

"Gregory is a male nurse she knew at Weathergill," he explained. "She brings him up during times of extreme stress. He was a calming influence during her worst periods there. I imagine she realized for the first time that she's in a hospital and called to him for help. I agree she probably should be started back on medication. It would be best if she can be moved to Psychiatry. Are you ready to release her from MICU?"

I was and I wasn't. I wanted her to go but I also wanted to monitor her heart another night, and cardiac monitoring is not available on the psychiatry ward.

Dr. Cohen recommended we begin Haldol, a major tranquilizer, and that she go to Psychiatry in the morning. I wrote the order: 1 mg Haldol intramuscularly every 12 hours.

Haldol worked and Judy calmed down. There was no more screaming and the following morning, July 6, she was transferred to Psychiatry.

Followup

Triavil was re-started on the Psychiatry ward but at a higher dose: 4-25. Judy's psychosis improved once again on medication and everyone was encouraged. Mrs. Bilowitz agreed to administer the medication at home and to keep the container locked away. Under this condition Judy was released at the end of July.

At home either her mother or the maid gave out the pill, twice a day, and watched Judy swallow it. Then the container was secured, a precaution taken only to prevent an impulsive drug overdose. There were of course other ways for someone in Judy's situation to attempt suicide.

The new dose worked well and Judy seemed to get better. She sometimes went shopping with her mother and on occasion took one-day trips with both parents. She even attended two meetings of the gardening society in the home of a family friend.

For most of August Judy was watched like a fragile child, but as she improved her parents' concern over another suicide attempt lessened. Dr. Cohen saw Judy regularly and did not find her overtly suicidal.

Judy mother and father so desperately wanted her to live a normal life. As time passed they more and more treated her like a responsible adult. There was even talk with Dr. Cohen of allowing Judy to self-administer the Triavil, though no decision had yet been made.

Judy must have been aware of this change in attitude. Was she just waiting and plotting another attempt? Or was her mind too disordered to make such plans? Whatever the thought processes in her head, one day in December of that same year Judy found the almost-full Triavil container sitting on the kitchen counter. Why and how it came to be left out, and for how long, we never learned. If Judy hesitated or pondered or fought the temptation, we'll never know. We do know that she opened the bottle and swallowed all the tablets, then threw the empty container in the trash and went to lie on her bed. This all happened about 11 a.m. Her mother was out shopping and the maid had the day off.

By supper time Judy Bilowitz was dead.

3. Medicine By Default

"You asked them WHAT?" My voice was raised in mock anger, to show the housestaff on morning rounds that Dr. Howard Stine's question was unacceptable. Shortly after admitting an 88 year-old man with pneumonia the intern had posed a certain question to the patient's son and daughter.

"I asked them," Dr Stine repeated, 'Do you want us to do everything for your father?' "

"And what did they say?"

"They said yes."

"I see." I waited a few seconds for someone to offer comment. Dr. Stine was far from the first neophyte physician to ask such a silly question, and he surely wouldn't be the last. Instead of responding, everyone on rounds — two interns, a senior resident, two nurses — looked past me in the direction of the patient, Jack Smilovsky. We were standing outside his room and sliding glass doors made him easily visible.

I knew what the housestaff were thinking. 'Well, it's probably not a good idea for Mr. Smilovsky to receive too much heroics, but if that's what his family wants, what are you going to do?'

"Barbara, what do you think of Howard's question?" Barbara Milo, the resident on the case, had rounded with me many times and knew my feeling about this recurring problem. Barbara is quick-witted and able to display the right amount of sarcasm when appropriate. Turning to Howard, with her head cocked slightly toward the patient, she went right to it.

"Do they want him dialyzed if his kidneys fail? Do we intubate him if his brain slips between his vertebrae? Do we send him for a heart transplant if he doesn't respond to drugs? Do we give platelet transfusions if his bone marrow goes zippo? Do we..."

"OK, Barbara, thank you." I looked toward Howard but spoke to everyone. "WE don't know everything that can be done. How can you ask a patent's family if THEY want everything done? Medical technology is endless, infinite!

"Soon we'll be sending patients into space, for god sakes, to treat them with zero gravity! Do the Smilovsky children want us to send their father into space? Did you ask them?" Everyone laughed. At least I had their attention. Dr. Stine was buried by the laughter but he managed to speak up.

"Dr. Martin, what should I have asked his family?"

"Not a zero option question. With what you asked, either they could say yes — as they did — or 'no, don't do everything.' But saying no puts them on an instant guilt trip. Maybe their understanding of 'don't do everything' is that we'd let him die for want of an aspirin or a bedpan. Who knows? You didn't give them any realistic options. It was like you came out and said: 'OK, we've got your father — does he live or die?' What *could* they say?

"Now that they've said yes, you've left Mr. Smilovsky open for mega technology. Maybe not the space shuttle — yet — but just about everything else. Look at him."

I slid open the doors and we went in and surrounded his bed. It was a pathetic scene. Mr. Smilovsky looked his age plus another ten years: gaunt, wasted, emaciated, out of touch with what was happening. His eyes were half closed and sunken into their orbits. His open mouth showed only toothless gums and a tongue that moved ceaselessly back and forth, without purpose. He might be suffering, but nothing in his eyes or hands or mouth communicated any feeling. This was not a human being so much as a heart and pair of lungs inside an ancient body. Mr. Smilovsky deserved antibiotics, a warm bed, and kindness. He did not deserve — because he would not benefit by — artificial life support.

At the start of rounds we learned that Mr. Smilovsky had been in Mt. Zion Nursing home for four years, the last two completely bedridden and demented from longstanding Alzheimer's disease. When he developed fever and shortness of breath he was sent to Memorial's emergency room. Lacking any clear directive about use of heroics the ER doctors sent him directly to MICU, where questions about how far to go were (apparently) first asked.

Now, at the seeming behest of his children, neither of whom, to be sure, had demanded anything in particular, we were obligated to do anything and everything to keep him alive. The medical diagnoses were pneumonia, sepsis, and dementia. Treatment was with antibiotics, fluids, and nasogastric feeding.

Mr. Smilovsky's condition was tenuous. Any hour he might 'need' an artificial ventilator for respiratory failure. An hour after that he might 'need' infusion of dopamine to support his blood pressure. Then he might 'need' a pacemaker, kidney dialysis, and a host of other readily available medical technologies.

For the moment however, his care looked reasonable; he had not yet entered the realm of high tech. I was ready to move on but the other intern on rounds, Pier Simpson, asked: "Aren't we obligated to do what's necessary? I mean, isn't that why he's here?"

Blessed be the intern who bids me to continue. Professional life would be lonely without someone to TEACH.

"Pier, how many people die each year in this country?"

The intern shrugged.

"Well, how many people are *in* this country. You need to know that piece of trivia first." After a few seconds of silence from Pier I said, "Anybody?"

"About two hundred and fifty million," said Molly, one of the nurses."

"Right. Now how many people die each year, of all causes?"

"About a million?"

"No, actually it's about two million. Now, excluding those who die before they can get to a hospital, and children, and accident victims, let's say that about one million mostly elderly people die of chronic disease or end-stage illness or old age. Furthermore, lets say they all end up in hospitals like Memorial, and that they all get connected to life support machines just as they are about to die."

"Dr. Martin," Molly interrupted. "Shouldn't we discuss this outside his room?" Actually, it didn't matter to Mr. Smilovsky, I was sure of that. But our proximity to the patient bothered Molly so I agreed to continue outside. We walked out and closed the sliding doors behind us.

"For the sake of argument, lets say that life support therapy prolongs each patient's dying by an average of two weeks. They will all die soon anyway, because that's the premise, but we're going to interfere with nature a little by instituting artificial ventilation, pressors, and any other life support deemed medically necessary. Furthermore, this is all going to be done in intensive care units like ours. How much are we talking about?"

As soon as conversation on rounds turns to economics everyone perks up and listens. It never fails. I now had their undiluted attention.

"It depends on what each hospital bill is," said one of the interns.

"Right. Let's say two weeks of therapy before each patient surrenders to nature — that seems about the average length of time ventilators can keep them going. Remember, they are destined to die anyway. Now the basic room rate is a thousand a day. Added to that are charges for antibiotics, respiratory care services, x-rays - tons of x-rays - and other odds and ends, roughly twelve hundred a day above the basic room rate. Twenty-two hundred a day is the average hospital charge for a MICU ventilator patient. It's a lot more if the patient is dialyzed or gets a pacemaker or has any surgery. Anyway, at fourteen days for the typical terminal ventilator patient, we're talking about a little over thirty thousand dollars each, and that's not counting professional fees.

"Some patients will last longer than two weeks, others will go quicker no matter what you do, but thirty thousand is probably a nice, conservative figure. Now, what's thirty thousand times one million?" A pocket calculator was brought out.

"Thirty billion dollars," said Dr. Stine, with some awe in his voice. The others just raised their eyebrows in acknowledgement. One nurse muttered "wow."

"That's right. Thirty billion dollars. Not the national budget, but not a small amount either. And for what? To prolong dying two weeks? It seems ridiculous, does't it? Fortunately, those one million patients don't all end up in our ICU or anyone else's. Many die at home, or in the nursing home, or even in the hospital, in a quiet room with their family and no tubes or machines."

"But you would save some of those patients," said Dr.

Simpson. "How can you decide ahead of time when it's inappropriate to be heroic?"

This intern is a jewel, I thought. He must round with me more often.

"That's right. Statistically some of them might *not* die. They might go on and *live* on the machines. Like Mrs. Jackson."

"Who is Mrs. Jackson?" asked Dr. Stine.

"Barbara, tell him."

"Mrs. Jackson is an 80-year-old demented woman who has been here about six months. She was only in MICU for two of those months. Now she's up on Tower North. We can't get her off the ventilator. And no nursing home will take her *and* her machine."

The two interns remained silent.

"Look, the whole point is," I continued, "doctors have to make decisions. Ideally, life and death decisions should be made with the input of the patient and family. Mrs. Jackson's family, as I recall, was never given an option about what to do. Now they're stuck and we're stuck. And Mrs. Jackson's stuck. Ask her if she's happy. She doesn't even know what planet she's on. Should we have to spend thirty billion dollars to keep one elderly, otherwise dying patient artificially alive?"

There was no answer. It was time to change course.

"Pier, would you intubate Mr. Smilovsky if he were ninety-eight?"

"Well, it depends on the circumstances." A beautiful hedge. No answer at all.

"How about a hundred and eight?"

"Maybe." Now I had Dr. Simpson on the defensive, and loosing ground.

"How about if he was one hundred and ten years old, and you had documented evidence of metastatic cancer to every major organ."

"No, of course not, Dr. Martin."

"So, you're willing to draw the line somewhere. But you feel uncomfortable about Mr. Smilovsky because he doesn't have widespread cancer. Only pneumonia and sepsis, theoretically treatable conditions. I understand that. At least you admit there is a line to draw."

Dr. Stine spoke up. "Dr. Martin, how would you have handled Mr. Smilovsky's family?"

"First of all, I wouldn't call it 'handling.' Explaining the situation is what you really want to do, in terms they can appreciate. I've never met relatives that want their mom or dad or sister or brother kept alive as a vegetable on a machine. Well, I take that back. We had one a few years ago, but the daughter had a few loose bolts, so that doesn't count; she could never understand the difference between near-brain-dead and sleeping. Sensible families *don't* want relatives kept alive on machines, with no hope of return to humanity. You have to discuss the situation in these terms.

"We should simply tell them the truth. 'Your father is eighty-eight. He's at life's end. Nothing we do will restore his mind or body to anything better than he was last week. The most we can hope to accomplish is a return to his former state, demented and bed-confined. If his breathing stops we're legally obligated to use machines to keep him going, unless you tell us otherwise. We'd obviously like to know his own wishes, but that's not possible, so I'm afraid it's up to you.'

"You'll be amazed at how often they will say, 'No, Dad wouldn't want that. Do what you can to make him comfortable, but no life-support machines.' Or, they might ask you for more information: 'What are his chances of getting off the machine once he's connected? What do you recommend? What would you do if this was your father?' The point is, you've established a dialogue and given the family realistic options. You can easily take it from there.

"If you get a clear sense that heroics and artificial life support are not to be used, you can order 'Do Not Resuscitate'; then, at least, everyone knows how far to go or not to go. If he's made 'DNR' we don't end up with a social service disaster like Mrs. Jackson."

*　　*　　*

Fortunately Mr. Smilovsky did not need artificial life support. He survived pneumonia and was sent back to his nursing home. But the man in the next room didn't fare as well.

Mr. Zigson was 82 when he came to our ICU. For Mr. Zigson everything *was* being done. By default. He received medicine's top technology not because he requested it, or his family demanded it, but because there was no one to call a halt.

Mr. Z had no relatives anyone knew about, only a legal guardian. In the nursing home he was thoroughly demented but not as bedridden as Mr. Smilovsky. He could sit and walk with assistance but had to be fed by nurses' aides.

Mr. Z was sent to Memorial Medical Center for impending kidney, heart and lung failure — about to die, in other words. His mind was too far gone to give insight into his own wishes for treatment. Having no family around (there were rumors of relatives in far away places, but we never saw any and no one ever called), we had to rely on his legal guardian, an attorney long ago appointed by the court.

The attorney's knowledge of Mr. Z's medical condition was close to zero. He preferred it this way "in order to stay objective and not bias myself." To help preserve this state of blissful ignorance he never visited Mr. Z in the hospital. When confronted over the phone, on the day of Mr. Z's admission, with the important questions — How far should we go? Can we make him DNR? What would Mr. Zigson want if he could tell us? — the attorney was non-committal: "Do what you have to do."

What did we have to do? Was it right to assault Mr. Z's body with tubes, needles, monitors, a ventilator and other assorted devices? Was it right to take over the function of his heart, lungs, kidneys, pancreas, and stomach without his consent? Was it right to feed his gut with food that never touched his tongue and replenish his blood with scarce blood products? Was it right *not* to do these things?

The ethical questions were weighty but the practical answer to all was simple: protect yourself against the threat of litigation. No one could fault you for trying to save his life, only for letting him die.

Having no one around to call a halt, physicians often must do things they feel are ethically or morally or socially wrong. If we let Mr. Z die a natural death (God forbid!) and his estate came up for probate, some long lost relative might come zinging out of the West to pursue an award commensurate with the charges — wrongful death, medical malpractice, mercy killing, *euthanasia.* (It's happened before.) Yet if he had a third cousin (or legal guardian) willing to say 'No, don't do this,' and that decision was consistent with our own sense of medical propriety, we could have stopped.

Mr. Z had no one, so we practiced medicine by default. And the default mode is *everything.* No one caring for Mr. Z thought it proper to begin artificial ventilation when his breathing failed. Artificial ventilation was begun without hesitation. No one felt comfortable about starting hemodialysis when his kidneys failed. He was dialyzed. And no one felt good about giving blood transfusions when his gut began to ooze the vital fluid. He was transfused.

When we consulted a surgeon to advise about the intestinal bleeding she did not operate, not because it was inappropriate (the guardian would have given permission), but because we were finally able to stem the bleeding with more conservative measures. "Call me if the bleeding resumes," she noted on the chart. She *would* have operated had it been necessary.

And when Mr. Z's heart began acting in strange ways — here a beat, there a beat, and frequently no beats for many seconds — the cardiologist didn't hesitate to place a pacemaker, "considering that everything possible is being done for this gentleman."

By day 14 of Mr. Z's stay in MICU — the same day I chided Dr. Stine for his 'do everything' question to the Smilovsky family — Mr. Z was fully hooked up, a vegetable artificially maintained by the best that medicine has to offer.

Through his mouth entered a foot-long, clear plastic endotracheal tube. Three-fourth's of the hollow tube lay in his mouth and trachea; the other quarter dangled outside his face and connected via plastic piping to the ventilator. Twenty-two times a minute the machine went Whoosh! (air in), swishhh (air out). Whoosh!-Swishhh, Whoosh!-Swishhh...

Another machine monitored blood pressure continuously via

a thin plastic catheter in his radial artery. A larger catheter invaded one of his neck veins, through which an infusion of dopamine helped maintain his blood pressure sufficient to perfuse kidneys and brain. A nasogastric feeding tube entered his nose and ended in the small intestine. A bladder catheter exiting his penis allowed urine to flow freely into a bag for easy collection. The latest and most expensive antibiotics went through another thin plastic catheter in his right forearm. A rectal tube helped funnel his diarrhea — a side effect of the antibiotics — into yet another plastic bag.

On rounds we discussed Mr. Z from head to toe, noting tubes, machines, drugs, diagnoses. I was satisfied that things were being handled correctly, and had very little to add. What more could one say? Everything was being done, practically every organ was supported by some drug or device. Altogether we counted seven tubes and catheters (tracheal, rectal, two intravenous, arterial, bladder, plus one for hemodialysis), three life support machines (ventilator, kidney dialysis, cardiac pacemaker), and 10 different drugs, including the blood-pressure-supporting dopamine. Whatever the outcome, the housestaff were on top of Mr. Z's care and the training program was being served.

Or was it? Each device or drug we used for Mr. Z is a major advance in medical therapy. Each, in its own way, has done wonders for patients. You can find many articles that show how each therapy has improved survival by some important percentage. For example, thousands of people are gainfully employed because of kidney dialysis, without which they would have died.

But were all these therapies *in toto* appropriate for Mr. Zigson? What is known about using multiple life support devices in elderly, demented patients? Do they help? Is there a point of no benefit, when the second or third or fourth machine will add nothing but expense and patient suffering?

Molly called it. "Dr. Martin, why are we doing all this?"

"We're caught, Molly. We have no choice. No one's taking responsibility for decisions about Mr. Z. We are in a legal conundrum."

The nurses and housestaff looked at me as if *I* should be

responsible, and I became a little defensive.

"*I* didn't order hemodialysis — Dr. G. started it (they knew this — I was pointing out the obvious). Dr. G. doesn't want to go on record withholding a life-saving therapy. We asked his opinion about what to do for the kidney failure. What else could he say? Dialyze!

"Ditto the cardiologist and everyone else. We're *all* responsible. The whole thing's absurd, but at least there's one consolation."

"What's that?"

"My second law of intensive care."

"Second law? What's your first law?"

"Don't you know?" They did not.

"Ok, the first law: If it happens here it happens everywhere. This kind of thing is going all over the country, every day."

"What's the second law?"

"Money not spent on dying patients will not go to feed hungry children."

*　*　*

The medical and moral travesty continued for another week. After that the dopamine infusion no longer worked and Mr. Z's blood pressure bottomed out. There was nothing else all our machines and chemicals could do. Nature won.

Mr. Z's total hospital bill came to $73,475.37. Not counting professional fees.

4. A Strange Pneumonia

One day in March 1985 — the year is important — we received a patient from another hospital: Reginald Herbert III, a 46-year-old oil company executive. In April of that year Mr. Herbert was hospitalized at a non-teaching suburban hospital with an undiagnosed and progressive lung infection. For two weeks his doctors tried in vain to diagnose the cause of infection, finally concluding that he needed an open lung biopsy.

An 'open' biopsy is a major operation, literally an opening up of the chest cavity to remove a piece of lung tissue. Mr. Herbert was transferred to our care mainly because Memorial Medical Center is better equipped for this procedure. He arrived on a Friday afternoon, in preparation for surgery the following Monday. On exam he was short of breath, breathing rapidly, and had a temperature of 102. He was "acutely ill" and could only talk with great effort because of respiratory distress. We obtained most of his medical history from the transfer records and Mrs. Herbert, a trim, fortyish woman who answered our questions but never went out of her way to volunteer more than was asked.

The facts were meager. Mr. Herbert had been well until three months before hospitalization, when he first noted onset of fatigue and a dry cough. Two seven-day courses of antibiotics, taken as an outpatient, did not change his symptoms.

Initially his outpatient chest x-ray was read as normal so pneumonia was not a tenable diagnosis. He soon became quite ill with high fever, sweats, and persistent dry cough, and at that point entered the suburban hospital where he underwent a battery of tests, including fiberoptic bronchoscopy. All test results were non-diagnostic. His white blood cell count was elevated and he had fever, cough and an abnormal chest exam, so pneumonia seemed a good possibility. Sure enough, a few days prior to transfer a shadow appeared on his chest x-ray and his physicians came to recommend the open lung biopsy.

Mr. Herbert's travel history fueled speculation of an exotic infection. As an oil company executive he had traveled to many countries, mostly to South America. Mrs. Herbert said he had spent about half of the previous two years abroad, in blocks of 6 to 8 weeks. She never went with him because they had two teenage kids in school.

Did he ever have pneumonia before? No, she said. Did he become ill on any of his overseas trips? Nothing that she knew about. Had either she or her children experienced any febrile illnesses in the previous year? No.

What an interesting case! Middle-aged executive with fever and pneumonia of uncommon cause. We ran through the "differential" of possible diagnoses and why he might not have responded to empiric antibiotic therapy. By the time of transfer Mr. Herbert had already received five different antibiotics, two as an outpatient and three more in the suburban hospital. Any common or typical infection should have been clobbered.

There was no evidence for the usual causes of pneumonia, such as Legionnaire's disease, mycoplasma, streptococcus, staphylococcus, and hemophilus. The one other infection that always has to be considered, tuberculosis, seemed unlikely; tests at the suburban hospital were negative for TB infection, both the TB skin test and a special bone marrow exam.

There is a 'waste basket' category of 'viral' pneumonia, often diagnosed only by excluding everything else. Viral infections are often hard to diagnose. They usually require checking blood samples weeks apart, and the blood has to be sent to a special state lab. We were not ready to call this a viral pneumonia.

There are many other diseases in the world alien to most Americans: malaria, schistosomiasis, blastomycosis, aspergillosis, tularemia, filariasis. Could Mr. Herbert have one of these exotic illnesses. Very possibly.

We also considered non-infectious problems like cancer, lupus erythematosus, and rheumatoid disease but these all seemed highly unlikely. Even AIDS was considered, though there was no history of homosexuality or drug abuse, the only associated risk factors known at the time. Even so, an AIDS antibody test was sent out prior to his transfer.

Whatever Mr. Herbert's diagnosis, we agreed with the need for the open lung biopsy; it just might reveal an unusual and treatable infection. Perhaps one out of a thousand pneumonia patients have to be taken this far to make a diagnosis.

*   *   *

Mr. Herbert went rapidly downhill. By Sunday evening his respiratory rate was very rapid, he was a bit confusional, and his blood oxygen tension was uncomfortably low. All signs pointed to impending respiratory failure. We intubated him and began artificial ventilation. Unless the lung biopsy showed a treatable pneumonia his prognosis for survival seemed poor.

He went to surgery Monday morning in critical condition: ventilator-dependent, breathing 100% oxygen, semi-comatose. The surgeon quickly opened his chest and excised a small piece of left lung. One half of the biopsy specimen went into a bottle of formalin for fixation and staining; thin slices of this piece would be examined under the microscope. The other piece went into a bottle of saline, for culture of bacteria and fungi.

Twenty minutes after the biopsy Mr. Herbert's chest was closed, save for a drainage tube that is routinely left in place. Mr. Herbert went to recovery and then, an hour later, was returned to MICU.

Unfortunately the effects of the operation, added to his debilitated state, made it impossible for him to breathe without the ventilator. We could not remove the endotracheal tube until he improved, and improvement would require a treatable diagnosis.

*   *   *

On Tuesday morning we had the answer. Mr. Herbert was suffering from *pneumocystis carinii* pneumonia, the commonest type of pneumonia in AIDS patients. Coincidentally, his AIDS antibody test returned from the lab the same day. It was positive.

The pieces fell rapidly into place. Our patient had a classic presentation for AIDS but his physicians, myself included, were somewhat fooled by his social background and our own inexperience with the disease at the time. How could an upper middle class executive have AIDS? In 1985?

But he did. And that is why none of the antibiotics had helped Mr. Herbert; he had not received drugs that attack *pneumocystis carinii*.   We immediately began the appropriate antibiotic, trimethoprim-sulfamethoxasole.

Because Mr. Herbert was in MICU, and I was available when the diagnosis became established, it fell to me to tell his wife. How to do it? There was no point in being coy or misleading, as that approach invariably backfires. I had told many patients and families terrible news but never, I realized, had a diagnosis of AIDS been that news.

I met Mrs. Herbert in the ICU on Tuesday afternoon as she was coming out of her husband's room. She was alone.

"We have the results of the biopsy," I said, matter-of-factly. She looked at me without responding, waiting for me to continue.

"It looks like it's (the truth wasn't so easy after all) the type of infection seen in AIDS patients."

I expected some expression of disbelief, or denial, or even anger, but she only said, "I see." If she was surprised at the diagnosis she didn't show it. This woman seemed like a rock. I hesitated to continue the discussion but continued.

"Also, the blood test sent out last week has just come back. It is positive for antibody to the AIDS virus."

In a most *un*inquisitive tone she responded: "I wonder how he got AIDS?"

I wondered with her. "Did he receive any blood transfusions in the last 5 years? The blood of AIDS carriers can infect otherwise healthy people."

"No, not to my knowledge," she said.

"He didn't use any drugs, did he?" I hoped she was not offended by this question.

"No, of course not," she said in a monotone, showing no offense but also no emotion. I thought it peculiar that she seemed so much more certain about drug abuse than about blood transfusions.

Suddenly it dawned on me. She *did* know how he got AIDS and she *wasn't* surprised at all. It now seemed awkward to ask the obvious question so I let it pass. In truth I was embarrassed to ask if Reginald Herbert III, father of her two children, was homosexual.

"Do you wish to be tested?," I asked.

"No, I don't think so. It's not necessary."

* * *

Over the next several days Mr. Herbert continued to do poorly. He did not respond to the antibiotic for *pneumocystis*, probably because it was begun too late or his infection was too far advanced. He remained ventilator-dependent and unresponsive.

Meanwhile, Mr. Herbert's family physician, who had followed him from the beginning of the illness, learned more about the Herberts and their marital relationship. The Herberts had not had sex together for over 18 months. His lack of interest, and some pictures of men Mrs. Herbert found in his suitcase, made her strongly suspect homosexuality. She presumed that much of his homosexual activity took place abroad. Mrs. Herbert denied all sexual activity since he left her bed. And she repeatedly declined to be tested for the AIDS virus.

Mr. Herbert continued to deteriorate and died seven days after the operation, of sepsis and respiratory failure. Mrs. Herbert did not grant permission for an autopsy.

Comment

By the end of 1981, the year AIDS was first reported, there were 281 known cases in the United States. By the middle of 1991 there were over 115,000 *deaths* from AIDS, including 31,196 AIDS deaths in 1990 alone.

Our hospital, unlike many teaching hospitals on the east and west coast, has not been inundated with AIDS patients. However, like every other hospital the number of AIDS patients we see has increased yearly over the past decade.

In the United States AIDS is still primarily a disease of young men, although AIDS is also becoming a leading cause of death among women. (For the past decade nine out of ten AIDS

deaths were men). Risk factors for AIDS include homosexual/
bisexual activity (59.1%), intravenous drug abuse (21%) and blood
transfusions (2.8%); the last group includes many hemophiliac
patients. Heterosexual activity accounts for about 4% of all AIDS
cases; the disease occurs from sexual contact with someone from
one of the other groups.

Fortunately, newer techniques for diagnosing *pneumocystis
carinii* pneumonia have obviated the need for open lung biopsy.
Now the diagnosis of PCP can usually be made right away, with
relatively little risk to the patient.   The diagnosis is often
established by instilling some saline into the lungs through a
flexible, fiberoptic bronchoscope, and suctioning the saline out a
few seconds later.   When these 'saline washings' are carefully
examined under the microscope they will almost always reveal the
pneumocystis organisms in patients who have PCP.

Pneumocystis carinii is the most common cause of pneumonia
in AIDS patients. With early diagnosis and aggressive antibiotic
therapy most AIDS patients recover from their first infection of
PCP. It is recurrent infections from opportunistic organisms like
pneumocystis that have caused most of the AIDS mortality.

5. Asthma in the Last Trimester

About five percent of the population in industrialized countries suffers from asthma. An asthma condition can range from minimal symptoms, with little or no impact on daily activities, to severe and life-threatening disability. Asthma can develop at any age. I have often seen asthma develop *for the first time over age 60* — and in people with and without an allergic history.

In an asthma attack smooth muscles lining the bronchial tubes, the airways of the lungs, contract or tighten. This contraction (also called bronchospasm) leads to narrowing of the airways. At the same time the bronchial walls become inflamed and secrete thick mucous into the airway, causing further narrowing. To gain some idea of what it feels like during a severe asthma attack, try breathing through a straw with your nose plugged. As you breathe gradually pinch the middle of the straw until it closes about half way. Now jog in place.

In people with asthma a variety of stimuli can bring on an attack of bronchospasm, including allergic reactions, upper respiratory infection (including the common cold), exercise, climatic changes, cigarette smoke, and emotional distress. Whatever the precipitating event the result is the same: ob-struction to air flow, wheezing, and a feeling of air hunger.

In a desperate attempt to bring in more air the asthmatic recruits 'accessory' breathing muscles (mainly in the neck and shoulders) and breathes faster. At the height of an asthma attack the patient looks like he (or she) just ran a marathon race (keep breathing through that pinched straw and you will too).

By definition asthma is *reversible* airways obstruction. The bronchospasm and excess mucous usually abate with appropriate medication. The operative word is 'usually.' Sometimes asthmatics don't respond to treatment, or respond so slowly that their condition requires hospitalization. Fortunately only a small percentage of asthmatics ever reach this stage.

*   *   *

Delores Buchanan was 24 when she came to the medical intensive care unit (MICU). Diagnosis: severe asthma, complicated by a 36-week pregnancy.

As a child Delores suffered from hay fever but not asthma. She received allergy desensitization shots from age 12 to 15. At 18, just out of high school, she first developed symptoms meriting the label of asthma: some wheezing and shortness of breath on exercise. These symptoms were controlled with oral and inhaled medication and over the next three years she never required hospitalization or emergency room treatment.

After a year of secretarial school she married and shortly afterwards became pregnant. There were no complications of her first pregnancy and at age 20 she delivered a healthy baby boy.

At 21 Delores suffered her first bad asthma attack. It started with a sinus infection. Nasal congestion progressed to mucous in her throat, cough, wheezing, dyspnea, more cough, more shortness of breath, and finally a trip to the doctor. Antibiotics and an asthma inhaler did not provide relief. Her shortness of breath progressed and she came to Memorial's emergency department. The severity of her symptoms mandated hospitalization for intravenous therapy, but she did not require intensive care. She gradually improved and was able to go home four days later, on a regimen of asthma inhalers and pills.

Her asthma remained quiescent for a while. At 22 she became pregnant again and delivered a healthy girl; she experienced no significant asthma symptoms, either during pregnancy or after delivery. While in the hospital she asked for and received one or two extra inhalation treatments but did not need intravenous asthma therapy.

After discharge Delores underwent thorough allergy evaluation. Multiple skin tests showed allergic responses to nothing more specific than dust and common mold. Desensitization shots were not recommended.   She continued regular visits to the allergy clinic and her asthma remained under control, with intermittent use of inhalers, for the next 18 months.

In 1987 she developed a severe asthma attack a few days after a head cold and was again hospitalized on the regular ward. After four days' therapy with intravenous medication she was discharged on a tapering course of prednisone (a corticosteroid, the most powerful anti-asthmatic medication). She continued to do well with outpatient therapy.

In the summer of 1988 Delores became pregnant for the third time. The first two trimesters were uneventful; she used an asthma inhaler as needed, about once every few days, and did not need prednisone. At 34 weeks gestation her asthma symptoms inexplicably worsened. She soon began inhaling asthma medication almost every day until things got so bad her husband brought her down to the hospital. Shortly after she arrived in the ED my beeper went off. I answered right away.

"Dr. Martin? Hi. This is Michael Highland, in the emergency room. I believe you know a patient who's down here, Delores Buchanan?" I had not seen her since the last hospital admission in 1987.

"I remember her. She's a young woman with asthma. What's happening now?"

"She's twenty-four-years-old and thirty-four-weeks pregnant, with one fairly severe asthma attack. I think she should be in MICU. She's not intubated but she's working very hard to breathe. We started her on methylprednisolone [an intravenous corticosteroid] and IV aminophylline [a bronchodilator]."

"Do you have a peak flow or blood gas?" I asked.

"Her peak flow is only about one hundred ten [liters/minute]. Let's see, I have her blood gas right here. PO-two is seventy-two, PCO-two thirty-eight, PH seven point four three. That's on room air." These results showed adequate oxygenation and ventilation, not a life-threatening situation. At least not yet. But then there was the fetus to worry about.

"Is her OB going to see her?"

"Yes. Dr. Senior's her obstetrician. His resident examined her and doesn't think she's in labor. They'll follow her in MICU but they think she's too sick for the OB floor."

"OK. Send her right up."

There is a rule about the course of asthma in pregnant patients: one third will improve, one third will have no significant patients: one third will improve, one third will have no significant change in symptoms, and one third will worsen. Unfortunately there is no way to predict which patient will end up in which group. Experience with an earlier pregnancy also doesn't predict what will happen.

There is also a simple rule for treating the pregnant asthmatic: treat the mother and the baby will be taken care of. If you don't treat the mother fully, for fear of harming the fetus, it can actually suffer from distress and hypoxemia.

Certain drugs, of course, should not be used during pregnancy. They include tetracycline (an antibiotic that stains fetal teeth); coumadin (a blood thinner that crosses the placenta); most newly-released drugs (not enough information to know about teratogenic effects); and any drug that might cause uterine contractions. This proscription still leaves available virtually all asthma drugs including corticosteroids, the most potent.

Mrs. Buchanan was put in room 5. After the nurses checked her weight and vital signs I went in. "Hello. I'm Dr. Martin." She nodded hello, smiled, and tried to look comfortable, but rapid breathing and contraction of neck muscles with each breath showed distress. Her face, full from pregnancy, displayed the fear and apprehension of severe asthma. Sweat covered her brow. Nostrils flared with each inspiration. Medication begun in the ER had helped a little but her respiratory rate remained fast, about 30 per minute. Also apparent were a distended belly poking up from beneath the bed sheet, legs swollen with edema fluid, and wheezing — audible without a stethoscope. In situations like this you don't walk in and ask, 'How are you?'

"Well," I said, "your asthma is beginning to respond to the medication. Just to be safe we'll keep you here until your asthma is better, then you can have that baby of yours."

"Good. . .I'm looking forward. . .to that." She could not speak more than a few words without pausing to catch her breath.

I ordered a chest X-ray to make sure we didn't miss pneumonia or some other acute problem. (A chest x-ray is safe, especially in the third trimester; as an extra precaution the mother's abdominal area is routinely shielded with a lead apron).

We inserted a catheter in her radial artery for frequent blood gas monitoring. An hour after arrival to MICU her respirations were still labored and arterial blood gases showed no major change. Not a bad sign, but not good either. Her chest x-ray was negative.

She received three basic asthma drugs: intravenous infusion of aminophylline and methylprednisolone, and inhaled albuterol via a nebulizer device every three hours. She also received oxygen through a nasal cannula. A cardiac monitor displayed her heart rate and rhythm, and a separate fetal heart monitor recorded her baby's heart rate. Mother's heart rate: 130 per minute, baby's 160. Both acceptable.

*   *   *

You're not supposed to die from asthma. After all, it's a reversible syndrome, there's good medication for it, every general physician is familiar with the symptoms and therapy. Yet year after year several thousand Americans do die from asthma *and the number is rising yearly*. Reasons for asthma deaths are varied. Over- and under-medication have both been blamed. Some patients are at fault for not seeking prompt medical attention. And, sadly, physicians are sometimes culpable for sending the patient home when he should be admitted to hospital. For about 15% of patients there is no explanation; they come for therapy on time, they get treated appropriately, but they just don't respond. Still, why the increase in deaths, especially with newer and more effective medications? No one knows for sure.

At Memorial we see about one death a year from pure asthma. In the case of Johnny Morgan, "see" is the appropriate word. He was young, poor, and unemployed. And he smoked. It was his additional misfortune to have bad asthma from the age of 15, asthma which, by the age of 21 had landed him in the hospital twelve times, four of them in intensive care.

The pity of Johnny Morgan's asthma is that each attack was fully reversible and probably preventable, at least in its severity. After a week of in-hospital treatment his lung function was normal or near normal. Then he would go home, smoke, catch a cold or develop bronchitis, and land in the emergency room.

Sixty-seven emergency room visits in six years, not counting the twelve that got him admitted to hospital.

Johnny was given countless regimens of tapering steroids, numberless asthma inhalers, and hours of instruction on how and when to use the medication. He was admonished about smoking so often that "tobacco addiction" came to be included in his list of discharge diagnoses.

The outcome was foretold in Mr. Morgan's outpatient clinic record, which included as many stamps of "NO SHOW" as followup notes by his clinic doctor. Two or three consecutive NO SHOW entries were followed by a cryptic "Adm. Hosp. - See Hosp. Chart."

In the middle of his 21st year, in June, Johnny developed progressive bronchospasm. His ever-present asthma inhaler did provide relief for a while but after several hours, perhaps longer, he began to feel that symptom of relentless suffocation that had brought him to our ED so often. A friend drove him to the hospital, about four miles distance on city streets. The ride over, as we learned later, was a nightmare for driver and patient. Johnny rapidly grew more distressed and his friend drove faster, running through red lights and stop signs, finally attracting a police car about half mile from the hospital. Johnny's friend stopped in front of the emergency room (he was familiar with the facility), got out of the car and ran to the officer who had pulled up behind. "My friend's not breathing!!"

The officer ran to the car, saw a slumped-over young man and began CPR in the front seat. The friend ran inside and yelled for help. Within seconds a first class, battle-ready, A-1 trauma team was at work on Johnny Morgan, his body spread out on the parking lot.

The ED team got him defibrillated, intubated, IV'd, infused, catheterized and medicated, but they couldn't get him ventilated. They were about two blocks too late. Johnny Morgan's lungs were beyond resuscitation and he died right there, 25 steps from doors marked "Memorial Hospital Emergency Department."

Autopsy revealed no illicit drugs or alcohol in his body, just the stiffest, most plugged-up lungs we have ever seen. A pure asthma death.

*   *   *

Whether from stress of pregnancy or severity of the attack, or both, Mrs. Buchanan did not improve. Her peak flow stayed between 80 and 150 liters per minute, about 20 to 30% of the predicted value. Arterial PO_2 remained safe at 70 to 90 but her CO_2 showed an ominous climb upward, to the mid-40s; in an acute asthma attack the higher the CO_2 the greater the severity.

The most severe asthmatics — patients with profound respiratory failure who are in imminent danger of asphyxiating — end up intubated and connected to a breathing machine (if they get to the hospital in time). Mrs. Buchanan was not at this stage but she was also not moving in the right direction.

On hospital day two we doubled her methylprednisolone dose (treat the mother) and started an antibiotic, erythromycin. We continued monitoring both maternal and fetal heart rate. Mother: 120; baby: 162.

The obstetricians saw Mrs. Buchanan twice a day. Their notes were terse and not generally helpful: "Not in labor. Baby OK. Continue current management."

"The baby's fine," Dr. Senior told me 48 hours into Mrs. Buchanan's unremitting asthma attack. "If you get her over this attack we'll let her go to term. Her due date is almost six weeks away. Just in case, I obtained permission for a C-section. How's she doing?"

"Not so great," I said. "The attack hasn't relented. What if she doesn't improve or gets worse? When would you want to do a C-section?"

"It's hard to say. There's a risk at thirty-four weeks. Also, if she suffered any hypoxemia during intubation it could be a real problem for the baby." He was right, of course. Surgery during a severe asthma attack can be a nightmare for mother and child. In addition, the baby would be born premature. Two strikes is no way to start out life.

By the afternoon of the third day she was clearly tiring out. Incessant dyspnea, muscle fatigue, and lack of sleep were taking their toll. Her peak flow was now consistently *below* 100 l/minute and the CO_2 level was almost 50! Blood oxygen was still

adequate but everything else pointed to one inescapable conclusion: Mrs. Buchanan's asthma attack would not relent until
she was delivered of child. I called Dr. Senior and gave him my
assessment.

"You could be right," he said. I knew I was right but he'd
have to make the final decision. "I'll be over in a few minutes to
see her."

Mrs. Buchanan didn't wait. Five minutes later she became
more fatigued and then suddenly *unarousable*. A 'stat' blood gas
confirmed the worst; she was severely acidotic from a buildup of
carbon dioxide. Treat the mother!

An anesthesiologist was called and within minutes Mrs.
Buchanan was intubated and connected to an artificial ventilator.
We had to give some IV sedation to coordinate her breathing
with the machine; it was that or risk losing the baby to maternal
distress.

Minutes after the intubation Dr. Senior arrived. He saw what
had transpired and immediately focused his concern on the baby.
"What happened to the fetal heart rate when she was intubated?"
he asked.

"Here, Dr. Senior." One of the nurse's handed him a long
paper strip, a continuous recording of the baby's heart rate. He
scanned the strip from beginning to end. For about 30 seconds,
just at the time of intubation, the baby's heart rate had fallen to
130 beats per minute, signifying a slight amount of fetal distress.
Now it was back up to 150. Sedation had apparently not caused
any major problem.

Turning toward me he said, "What do you think?"

"I think the baby's got to come out. We've given her
everything and she's going nowhere. Her lungs are tighter than
on the day of admission. She's in profound respiratory failure.
I think we got to her just in time with the ventilator. I
recommend C-section if it's at all possible." I knew it was
possible, I just wanted him to make the decision. I don't like to
force the hand of any surgeon.

"It's possible, just risky."

I pointed to Mrs. Buchanan. "True. But this is riskier.
Besides, shouldn't a C-section be safer now that we can control

her breathing?"

"Sure, but the baby will be born premature and could suffer more distress. Of course there's also the risk of leaving him in there. What's the mother's P-O-two?" he asked.

"One twenty. That's on forty percent oxygen."

He thought for a few seconds then announced. "We'll do it. You'll take her back afterwards?"

"No problem. She belongs here. You get to keep the baby."

We went out together to speak with Mr. Buchanan about the emergency C-section. A factory worker in his late 20s, he still had on his blue work clothes and steel-toed shoes. We explained the situation, the risks both ways, the worst that could happen if we did and didn't operate. He was in a state of bewilderment and left the decision in our hands, essentially reaffirming his earlier permission for the C-section.

Dr. Senior next placed a call to the head of neonatology, activating the hospital's protocol for high risk delivery. An hour later Mrs. Buchanan left MICU en route to Labor and Delivery, a floor above MICU. Safe transport required a team of four nurses and technicians: two to handle the cart, one to breathe her manually with an Ambu bag, and one watch the maternal and cardiac monitors.

Once in the delivery suite Dr. Senior and the anesthesiologist became responsible for her care. I went along as an observer, and to help in any way necessary.

$$*\quad*\quad*$$

"This lady is tight," said Dr. Kazeem, the anesthesiologist, "she's requiring a lot of ventilator pressure." I. T. Kazeem, a short, balding man in his 50s whom I have seldom seen dressed in anything but green surgical, has probably given more high risk anesthetics than anyone in the city. Seeing him in L&D did a lot to ease my own anxiety. His comment was also a question: were we doing everything possible for Mrs. Buchanan's asthma?

"I know," I said. "She's on maximal steroids, the works. The baby's got to come out before she'll improve."

Dr. Kazeem turned his attention to the surgeon. "How quick

are you, Dr. Senior?" A gentle reminder that speed was of the essence.

"Can you give me ten minutes of good anesthesia?" Dr. Senior replied.

"I can if her blood pressure holds up. I'm going to give her one hundred percent oxygen."

"The baby'll love it," responded Dr. Senior. "He's already high on aminophylline. Fetal heart rate?"

"One sixty and holding steady," replied a nurse.

"Scalpel."

"Retractors."

"Move than light a little bit down her abdomen. That's better. Hold it."

The dialogue sounded like some sort of Grade B movie. Only it was authentic, the patient's life *was* in balance, and our sweat under the hot ceiling lights was all too real.

"Mother's pressure is one hundred systolic. How're you doing with her belly?" Dr. Kazeem was sitting at Mrs. Buchanan's head and could not easily view the operation. I, on the other hand, could see both Dr. Kazeem and the operative field.

"I'm getting there," Dr. Senior replied. He was assisted by a third-year obstetrics resident and two scrub nurses. Between them I could see the incision. A wide low swath above her pubic bone exposed the distended uterus. Next Dr. Senior had to cut the uterine muscle. Slice. Slice. So easy in skilled hands. Be careful, a baby's in there! He cut some more and the abdominal muscles parted. Two hands disappeared into the cavernous sac. Ten seconds later the hands came out holding a pink baby — a girl. With one free hand Dr. Senior suctioned her mouth.

"Whaaaaaaa! Whaaaaaaa!"

Success. He handed her over to the neonatologist.

"How's mother doing?" Dr. Senior asked, ever so calmly.

"Holding steady. Sew her up," said Dr. Kazeem, relieved that one of his two patients was free and clear. I shared the relief. We all did. Whatever happened to Mrs. Buchanan, her premature infant entered life with an excellent chance of survival.

"She weighs twenty-two hundred grams. A little slow in reflexes," said the neonatologist. "Apgar is seven. I think she'll be all right. We'll keep her in NICU [neonatal intensive care unit] for a few days."

I walked over to view the crying infant. She looked fine to me, just a little small. I returned to the operating table and slipped my stethoscope under the drapes, to auscultate Mrs. Buchanan's mechanically-ventilated lungs. Still wheezing, still tight.

*   *   *

I was right. Despite the pain of a hysterectomy incision Mrs. Buchanan began to respond to our drugs. Rapidly. Within 36 hours we were able to extubate and disconnect her from the ventilator. She still wheezed, and her asthma attack was far from over, but recovery was now just a matter of time.

Her first post-extubation words: "When can I see my baby?"

"Soon, very soon. We can't bring Abigale to MICU because she might catch something. And you can't go to her until we're sure you're stable. We'll watch you a few more hours, then take you to her room." Mother and baby were reunited that evening. Breast feeding was out of the question but with some help Mrs. Buchanan bottle-fed and changed a diaper. The next day we transferred her out of MICU, to the OB ward, where her asthma continued to improve. As for Abigale, despite prematurity she developed no major complications. She went home seven days after birth, in the arms of her mother.

Comment

Mrs. Buchanan decided to have no more children and underwent tubal ligation. Her asthma continues to be easily controlled with pills and inhaled medication. As for Abigale Buchanan, she is growing normally and shows no signs of asthma.

6. "We can't kill your mother!"

As an intensive care doctor I've dealt with many ethical dilemmas, most involving decisions to start or stop artificial ventilation. One of the most difficult was that of Mrs. Virginia Tyson, an 80-year-old nursing home resident admitted to the medical intensive care unit April 27, 1989.

A month earlier she had fallen and fractured her right hip. She underwent a hip repair and returned to the nursing home, but had not walked since. Additional diagnoses were rheumatoid arthritis, emphysema, and cardiac disease. Dehydration, on top of her bed-confined state and chronic lung disease, led to acute respiratory failure. Shortly after arrival to MICU we had to place an endotracheal tube through her mouth and begin artificial ventilation.

The severity of her condition made it impossible to remove the tube and discontinue the machine ventilation. Although her acute medical problems were eventually corrected she could not be disconnected from the ventilator; each attempt led to severe shortness of breath. On May 4 she underwent tracheostomy, a procedure that places a short plastic breathing tube through an opening in the neck, allowing the larger and more uncomfortable mouth tube to be removed.

With tracheostomy a patient can eat while receiving artificial ventilation. The 'trach' tube is also much easier to care for than a mouth tube, and can remain in place indefinitely.

Mrs. Tyson's need for artificial ventilation did not improve after tracheostomy. She simply did not have the strength to sustain breathing without the machine.

Her closest family was two daughters, one of whom lived in a nearby state and the other far away, in Seattle. The nearby daughter stayed in town and visited her mother daily, and was in phone contact with her sister.

Mrs. Tyson remained mentally alert. She could not talk with the tracheostomy but was able to communicate with a pad and pencil. SIT ME UP. IS MY DAUGHTER HERE? MY THROAT IS SORE.

Reflecting a trait I've noted among the elderly in MICU, Mrs. Tyson never asked about her disease or prognosis. "We're trying to get you off the breathing machine," we told her often; she always nodded in appreciation but didn't raise any questions. She also never objected to the care we gave her.

I met with the daughter almost daily. A thin, pleasant woman, she was quite understanding about her mother's lack of progress. She never challenged what we were doing, and only asked that "mother be made comfortable." I felt no communication barrier between us, and also saw none between her and the MICU nurses.

Considering Mrs. Tyson's age, chronic illnesses, and ventilator-dependency, we raised the question of additional life support should other organs fail. Mrs. Tyson and her daughter requested no further life support or resuscitative measures, and a 'Do Not Resuscitate' order was entered in her chart.

No other organs failed and her lung condition did not improve. She remained stable, albeit ventilator-dependent. Our hospital allows for stable ventilator patients to go to a regular ward, so on May 9 we transferred Mrs. Tyson out of MICU.

At the request of Mrs. Tyson's internist I continued to follow her on the ward, and made another attempt to wean her from the ventilator shortly after transfer. When this failed I suggested that social service look for a nursing home that would take ventilator-dependent patients. Mrs. Tyson's original nursing home could not accept her back with the ventilator.

No matter how routine ventilators become for a hospital they are never routine anyplace else. In 1989 only two nursing homes in our metropolitan area accepted ventilator-dependent patients and they were both full. Still, we had no choice but to look for placement of Mrs. Tyson in a chronic care facility. She could not come off the machine without dying.

Attached to the machine she could in theory live many more years, although a sudden event, such as pulmonary embolism (blood clot in the lungs), could also end her life quickly. Her DNR status meant that we would not intervene if another bodily system failed, but it did not change the day-to-day care she needed and received. I felt sorry for Mrs. Tyson and her daughter, but there was nothing more we could do except continue medical care and attempt placement.

On May 15 I got a call from the resident caring for Mrs. Tyson. "Her other daughter is here and wants us to turn the ventilator off. She says her mother wants to die."

"I'll be right up."

In a few minutes I met this daughter, standing alone outside her mother's room The older of the two children, she appeared to be in her late 40's, physically similar but more aristocratic in bearing than her sister. As to temperament they seemed totally different. The Seattle daughter had only arrived that day, but wasted no time in getting down to business: "Dr. Martin, I want Mother disconnected from the ventilator."

"What? Your mother can't live off the ventilator."

"I know that. I know what I'm asking."

She had already learned about our failure to remove the ventilator. Calmly, I expressed amazement at her demand.

"Why all of a sudden?"

"Doctor it's *not* all of a sudden. Mother has always expressed her wish to die instead of being connected to a machine."

"But I've cared for your mother for three weeks. Neither she nor your sister said anything about turning the machine off."

"Did you ever ask them?"

"No, it never came up. We made her DNR, that was your mother's wish. But you're asking something totally different. If your mother had refused artificial ventilation before we began, it could have been withheld. Mentally competent patients have every right to make such decisions. But neither your mother or sister ever made that decision. What you're asking now doesn't make sense."

"I'm telling you what Mother wishes. My sister was just too timid to bring it up."

'Wow!' I thought. There's something strange going on here. What, I didn't know, but it got stranger.

"Let's go ask Mother now," she said. In disbelief I followed her into Mrs. Tyson's room.

There was no introduction to the subject. Not even, 'Mom, I brought the doctor in to discuss this matter.' Instead:

"Mother. Do you want to die?"

Mrs. Tyson nodded yes. There was no emotion to the nod. Just a dutiful yes.

"See," said her daughter. "Now will you disconnect the ventilator?"

It was time to be more forceful. I had a tough and determined woman on my hands. "Could I speak to you outside?" She agreed and we left Mrs. Tyson's room.

"I'm sorry but I cannot disconnect the machine. I respect your wishes and am not going to ignore your request. But I'm not the only one caring for your mother. This will have to be discussed with other physicians and the hospital's attorney. You have to understand, what you're asking has never been done before in this hospital. There is no way any single physician or nurse can just go in and disconnect a ventilator. We can't just walk in and kill your mother!"

"I'm *not* asking you to kill my mother. I'm only asking you to let her die a natural death."

"I know that's the way you see it. But you have to look at it from our perspective."

"When can you call these other physicians and the attorney? I want to get this resolved as soon as possible. Mother's suffered enough."

"How long will you be here this afternoon?" It was one o'clock.

"I'll stay as long as necessary."

"OK. I'll make some phone calls and see what I can arrange."

I called the chairman of our ethics committee (of which I am also a member) and explained the situation; he agreed to meet the next day, at noon. I then called the hospital attorney and outlined my understanding of the legal issues; she also agreed to the meeting. The nurses, social worker, and medical housestaff caring for Mrs. Tyson were also informed, and by 3 p.m. I had everything lined up.

I returned to the ward. This time both daughters were there. Somewhat to my surprise, the younger daughter expressed total agreement with her Seattle sibling, but also admitted to being "not very good at verbalizing Mother's wishes." Verbalizing? She hadn't ever *suggested* what now seemed written in stone.

"Are you sure your mother wants to die?"

"Oh, yes. Mother told me that many times. She's said that for years. She just never got a chance to say it here." Her tone was unsettling, almost accusatory. I was glad a meeting was arranged for the next day. Let others here this.

"Now," challenged the lady from Washington state, "will you disconnect Mother from the machine?"

"I already told you that's impossible for me to do. I've spent the last two hours arranging a meeting for tomorrow, at noon. Our lawyer and the chairman of the ethics committee will be there. Is that time OK?"

"Yes. We'll bring our family lawyer."

* * *

The next morning I came to see Mrs. Tyson on rounds and was immediately confronted by the head nurse.

"Mrs. Tyson's daughters were here last night. They were asking the night shift why Mrs. Tyson was being tortured, and why she can't be disconnected from the ventilator. Mrs. Tyson even wrote a note asking to be disconnected. The nurses are really feeling strained by their attitude. What are you going to do?"

I reminded her of the meeting and left it at that. Clearly, this issue had to be resolved quickly. I took some comfort in realizing that, having called the meeting, the decision was now out of my hands.

There were 12 people at the noon meeting, held in a library off the ward: 9 from the hospital staff, plus Mrs. Tyson's daughters and their attorney. I adopted the role of moderator, to both provide medical background and make sure the daughters' wish was fairly presented. It was also important that everyone understand the background against which such an extraordinary request was being made.

After introductions I briefly presented Mrs. Tyson's medical history, emphasizing that at no time did she or her younger daughter ask for the ventilator to be turned off. I explained how she was made DNR, and that this did not translate into disconnecting the ventilator in an awake patient under any circumstances.

I also explained how, because of emphysema and other medical problems, her lungs were damaged beyond repair, and that I saw no prospect for her living without the ventilator. I offered my best medical judgment that without the machine she would die within 24 hours.

Then, looking at the older sister I commented that "we were all surprised when you showed up and asked to have her machine disconnected."

I was not asking for a response but she volunteered one: "I'm truly sorry I didn't come earlier, but it was impossible. I am now here to see that Mother's wish is granted."

Looking toward the younger daughter I remarked, "I understand you are in agreement with this request?"

"Not only am I in agreement, it's what Mother wants. It's what we want. It's what should be done!" What conviction. Where had she been the last three weeks?

The floor was open for discussion. The night nurse on the ward spoke first. "Mrs. Tyson wrote me this note last night." The note was passed around. I had not seen it before. The ethics chairman suggested I read it out loud.

"'Please let me die. I don't want to go on living this way. Virginia Tyson.' Was either daughter present when she wrote this note?," I asked.

"No. Both had left the hospital."

The older daughter spoke up. "Look, I know this must seem strange to all of you, but you people don't *know* my mother. She never wanted to live like this. Mr. Barnes, the family lawyer, has known Mom for 40 years." She turned to the elderly gentleman, at least as old as Mrs. Tyson.

"That's true," he affirmed in a creaky, barely audible voice. She told me many times not to let this happen." (Why had none of this been made clear prior to admission?)

The ethicist spoke up. "I'm Dr. Knowles. I was asked to come because I head the hospital's ethics committee. I don't know your mother and have not cared for her, but I'm a physician and have cared for many patients in similar circumstances, that is elderly patients connected to a ventilator.

"I think I understand what you're asking. One problem we're all having — at least something that bothers me — is how this has developed. You are absolutely correct. The patient has a right to determine her destiny. The problem, from a purely ethical and moral perspective, is what is her real wish? I don't doubt for an instant your sincerity. It's just that I'm having trouble separating your mother's true desire from what she may be expressing out of guilt, perhaps for what her illness is doing to the two of you."

There! He said what we were all only wondering. Was Mrs. Tyson asking to die so as not to be a burden on her daughters — especially the older one, for whom the constraints of time, if not distance, seemed more of a problem than the younger daughter? Or were the sisters merely conveying what was truly their mother's wish from the very beginning?

Mr. Barnes objected. "That's not true. Mrs. Tyson has always said she didn't want to live like this."

Dr. Knowles responded. "I don't doubt that, Mr. Barnes. And I'm truly respectful of the awful situation she's in. I don't think any of us would want to live under these circumstances. I'm just expressing why we're all so surprised, and why it's difficult to accept what you are asking. If she had made this wish clear from day one, and the family agreed, then I think ethically there would be less confusion on the issue. I'm not saying we'd take her off the machine even then. It's just that, from an ethical viewpoint, the request would seem less unreasonable."

"Are you saying you won't take my mother off the machine?" asked the older daughter indignantly. Good, I thought; let everyone see what I've been up against.

It was our lawyer's turn to speak. A former RN, she was compassionate and direct. "First, let me say that I understand your request. I really do. I know your mother has no chance of getting off the ventilator, and I accept that it may be her wish to die rather than go on living this way. The truth is, under state law we can't disconnect the ventilator. Your mother is awake and alert, and we can't do anything that will lead directly to her death."

"You mean I'll need a court order to stop the machine?"

"Yes, I'm afraid so. I must warn you, though, that no court in this state has ever granted such a request on an awake patient. And if one did, we'd appeal it. Also, I don't think there's anyone in this room who would personally disconnect your mother's machine."

"Speaking for myself," I said, "as one of her physicians I could not disconnect the machine and watch her die, court order or not. Would any of the nurses be able to do it?"

The three nurses in the room quickly shook their heads and the discussion was over. Mrs. Tyson's daughters had presented their demand, entirely reasonable in their eyes, but unreasonable from a legal and ethical perspective. The daughters had lost the first round but they were prepared for the outcome.

Without missing a beat the older daughter said: "Then we'll take mother home."

*   *   *

Over the next several days prodigious arrangements were made to transfer Mrs. Tyson to the home of a local relative. We made it clear to the daughters that she could not be released until we felt assured she would receive adequate care. Sending ventilator-dependent patients home is not impossible and we have done it before. It just takes a lot of planning and some commitment on the part of the family.

The hospital's attorney felt that we could not block Mrs. Tyson's discharge unless we had evidence that the daughters might harm her. We had no such evidence. In fact both daughters were accepting of our decision not to disconnect the ventilator, coming as it did from such a powerful show of force and determination. They cooperated with all the people involved in the discharge, including respiratory therapists, visiting nurses, and Mrs. Tyson's social worker. Arrangements to send a ventilator patient home ordinarily take at least a week, and they did not try to rush us.

On the evening of May 21, four days after our meeting, Mrs. Tyson was found dead in bed. Her daughters had not been there for several hours, and the previous nurse check, only an hour earlier, had found the patient weak but otherwise stable. Her death was deemed due to natural causes. No autopsy was performed.

Comment

What Mrs. Tyson's daughters asked for was tantamount to active euthanasia. The ethical and legal perspective with which we confronted their wish is clearly stated in a position paper published by the American College of Physicians: "Although a patient may refuse a medical intervention and the physician may comply with this refusal, the physician must never intentionally and directly cause death or assist a patient to commit suicide. Active euthanasia remains illegal in all jurisdictions of the United States. Even if legalized, however, such an action would violate the ethical standards of medical practice." (American College of Physicians Ethics Manual. Annals Internal Medicine, August 15, 1989, Volume 111, page 334.)

7. The Yellow Man

Willie Duncan's body was a mess, the end result of a pint of whisky a day for God knows how many years. He was only 38 but looked 60.

When most people think of end stage alcoholics the visual image is probably one portrayed by Hollywood: a drunk stumbling down the street, or sleeping on a bar stool, or beating his wife, or abandoning her children for the bottle. The theater is also a source of impressions, for example the character of Eugene O'Neill's alcoholic mother in his autobiographical "Long Day's Journey Into Night."

Stage or screen, the portrayal is usually focused on the alcoholic's *behavior*: out of control, irrational, or self-destructive. But what about the *body*? Has Hollywood ever presented for our entertainment the physical persona of the terminal alcoholic? Hardly, and with good reason.

Maybe you'll see a closeup of a face just before the drunk slips into alcoholic stupor: grizzly beard, red lips, bloodshot eyes. And perhaps you'll hear some well-rehearsed lines: "I don't care — burp! — if you leave me — burp! — Give me a drink — burp!" ...fade away.

Movies — and television, for that matter — should not be faulted for glossing over the true clinical picture. In many cases it's too unpleasant, too *gory*. The kids might love it if the alcoholic was also a werewolf or vampire, but kids aren't interested in the last throes of an ordinary drunk.

You could go into any teaching hospital in America and find a patient like our Willie Duncan. He's yellow, head to toe; the eyeballs give it away. Normally white, Willie's eyes were a deep, obvious yellow, the result of liver failure and accumulation of yellow-tinged bile.

End-stage alcoholics have arms and legs thinned by malnutrition. Examine the skin in the forearms and you'll likely see purple blotches, the result of fragile capillaries and easy bruising. Take the bed covers off and you may find a distended, tense belly, like that of a child with kwashiorkor. The physiology is the same — massive fluid buildup due to lack of protein — but victims of kwashiorkor are starved for protein; in alcoholics the liver is destroyed by drink and can't make any.

Looking up from the beach ball belly you will often find a chest covered with red "spiders," superficial blood vessels in a star burst pattern about an inch in diameter. Press the center of one 'spider' and it will blanch; let go and it will fill quickly with blood from the center outward. These abnormal vessel clusters, called 'spider angiomata,' are another sign of severe liver failure.

The mind of the typical yellow man will likely be slipping away. Our Willie Duncan was confused and disoriented. He did not know the day, the date, or the president (end-stage alcoholics older than Willie often answer "Roosevelt" or "Eisenhower"). Even when you think the terminal alcoholic is lucid, he is not. Ask him to count back from a hundred by sevens (100...93...86... 79...); he can't do it.

There's more. Search carefully and you'll discover that the patient is bleeding internally. As the liver shrinks from the effects of alcohol the veins inside the esophagus — the tube connecting mouth to stomach — becomes engorged with blood. Normally, esophageal veins route their blood through the liver. The more the liver shrinks the more these veins distend until, like a balloon continuously filled with air, they burst open and spill blood into the esophagus. The dark red blood is both vomited up and passed in the stool, where it appears as mahogany-colored diarrhea.

Even if you've seen the Willie Duncans of America before, you will stare in amazement each time another yellow, bloated, bleeding patient comes to the hospital. It is a startling spectacle.

Not that our Willie Duncan wasn't forewarned. He was now in for his seventh hospital admission in as many years. Long before alcohol turned his liver into a rock hard lump of scar tissue Willie was told what to expect if he didn't stop drinking. During every hospitalization he was advised, cajoled, threatened: stop drinking.

In the early days he had a wife, a brother and sister; his relatives were told to get Willie to stop drinking or he would die from liver failure. Eventually his wife left him (or him her, it isn't clear which). Willie's brother was killed in a fight, leaving only a sister as immediate family. He had no children.

Nothing worked for Willie. Like most terminal alcoholics, Willie was poor. He had once held a steady job as a cab driver but was now on welfare and living with his sister. There was certainly no money for an expensive alcohol treatment program even if he were motivated to join one. His sister once persuaded him to enter Alcoholics Anonymous; he attended meetings only a few months before the bottle lured him away.

Willie's case reflected a sad fact: it is far easier to convince patients to go on a diet, exercise, or quit smoking, than to stop drinking. Alcoholism is a certifiable and often incurable *disease*. Except for a few specialized centers, most of which are expensive and closed to the uninsured, medical treatment is relegated to the *effects* of alcohol and not to the addiction itself.

In truth, Willie Duncan's alcoholism was as untreatable as terminal cancer. Willie Duncan came to MICU to die. The method chosen by his body was exsanguination. He was admitted one day in June with massive gastrointestinal bleeding.

In MICU we estimated that his engorged esophageal veins oozed blood at a rate of about 200 cc's an hour. Without some intervention his body would be empty of blood in 24 hours. Long before that he would die of shock.

Everyone in MICU knew Willie was terminally ill. But only 38 years old! How could we let him just bleed out? Doctors don't like to watch people bleed to death, even if therapy appears futile. We had to try something. We tried everything.

First we replaced his blood. In the first 48 hours he received eight units of blood and two units of fresh frozen plasma. Shortly after admission, during his first blood transfusion, gastro-enterologists passed a flexible scope (a procedure called 'endoscopy') into Willie's gut to identify the sites of bleeding.

As expected, the gastroenterologists found bleeding esophageal veins. (In addition to engorged esophageal veins alcoholics can also bleed from stomach and intestinal ulcers. Ulcer bleeding occurs from erosion into an *artery*. Esophageal bleeding is from a leaky or ruptured *vein*. The two causes of bleeding are treated differently.) His bleeding veins were injected, through the endoscope, with a latex material.

Endoscopic latex injection stops hemorrhage by changing the free-flowing venous blood into a harmless clot but the technique works only about 60% of the time. Initially it seemed to work for Willie then, five hours later, he vomited up about 100 cc's of dark red blood.

The next therapy tried was intravenous 'vasopressin', a potent vasoconstrictor. Vasopressin has long been used to control bleeding from the gastrointestinal tract. For stomach and intestinal bleeding the vasopressin must be infused directly into the bleeding artery. This intra-*arterial* infusion requires threading a long catheter through the thigh artery and then into the bleeding vessel itself, a highly invasive and specialized technique.

For bleeding esophageal veins — alone among causes of bleeding within the gastrointestinal tract — vasopressin works just as well when infused through a peripheral arm vein. We began Willie on 0.4 units of vasopressin per minute through an arm vein.

For the next 12 hours he was stable: no bleeding. Then he retched, leaned over the side of the bed and vomited up several hundred cc's of dark blood.

The gastroenterologists were summoned. What to do now? Surgery was not a viable option. No good operation exists for bleeding esophageal veins and Willie would not have survived surgery in any case. There seemed but one more thing to try: a Sengstaken-Blakemore tube. This three-foot long, hollow tube was introduced in the 1950s and named after the inventing surgeons. Once the main form of treatment for massive esophageal bleeding, the S-B tube is now used only as a last resort, when latex injection and vasopressin infusion fail.

The S-B tube is affixed at one end with two inflatable balloons, one for the esophagus and a smaller balloon for the stomach. When inflated with air, the esophageal balloon forces pressure against the hemorrhaging veins, much as you might stop bleeding from a cut by applying pressure. The esophageal balloon is basically a mechanical technique whose success depends greatly on proper positioning and the right amount of pressure.

To prevent the inflated balloons from moving and dislodging, the outside end of the S-B tube must be attached to a fixed object. Years ago the outside part of the S-B tube was taped to the patient's forehead but the tape always peeled off when the patient was moved. Then someone had a brilliant idea: use a football helmet. An S-B tube tied to the face mask of a football helmet works beautifully. End-stage alcoholics with esophageal bleeding all wear football helmets in the ICU!

An S-B tube was placed into Willie's stomach and the balloons inflated. Amazingly, the bleeding stopped. But what a sight! A thin, emaciated, disoriented yellow man with giant belly. Wearing a football helmet emblazoned with the emblem of our city's professional team. For two days Willie Duncan lay like a wounded linebacker, the bleeding stemmed by fragile balloons pressed against his gut.

Jokes are inevitable about such patients. "Willie's trying out for the team — at the rate they're going, he'll make first string." "I just got a call from [the coach]. He wants to see Willie right away. Let's clean him up." "Willie should try out; he won't hurt their chances for the superbowl." That year, our team and Willie Duncan were losers.

(Jokes are a necessary valve for ICU staff. We never really laugh at patients. We laugh at situations, at circumstances, at the human condition, and at ourselves. It is a healthy laughter.)

Six different doctors became involved in Willie's care this time around. If you asked each doctor what he or she honestly thought about his chances, none would admit to any optimism. I don't believe anyone held out much hope for Willie. I know I didn't, but still we tried. Was it inappropriate to do so? Should we have quit because Willie was an incorrigible alcoholic?

Given his age, I don't think so. The last thing you want to do is let a patient's lifestyle influence your care. It would be ethically wrong to limit care *because* he was an alcoholic. Once you start making that type of judgment you are on a very slippery slope. It is then only a small step to withholding care because someone smokes cigarettes, or eats too much, or doesn't get enough exercise, or drives a foreign car.

The only justification for holding back is if what you have to offer will not help, cannot help the patient. It is as morally wrong to offer treatment that cannot benefit the patient as it is to withhold treatment that may. Not being a specialist in esophageal bleeding and liver failure, I didn't want to make any life and death decision on Willie Duncan. If the gastroenterologists wanted to try multiple latex injections and ten S-B tubes (or surgery, for that matter) I could not legitimately object. Only the most experienced physicians should say there is nothing more to offer a dying patient.

Two days after the S-B tube was placed Willie's vessels opened up. Blood gushed everywhere. Dark red blood oozed out and around the S-B tube. Beneath his buttocks lay a puddle of mahogany-colored diarrheal stool. Before another unit of fresh blood could be infused Willie's heart stopped beating. Willie Duncan bled to death.

Comment

We obtained permission for an autopsy from Mr. Duncan's sister. At autopsy his liver was markedly shrunken to only about half its normal weight. His esophageal veins were enormous, over two inches across. One vein had a large rent down the side, the site of his fatal bleed. There was no evidence for cancer or infection.

In 1990 chronic liver disease was the ninth leading cause of death, claiming 26,000 lives. Many of these liver disease victims — like Willie Duncan — succumbed to the effects of chronic alcoholism.

8. Adult Respiratory Distress

Joe Woodbury, 35 years old, was healthy until January 11, 1982, when he developed a scratchy sore throat, no different in character or intensity from what many of us suffer every year. Even in retrospect, those early symptoms suggested nothing more sinister than a minor upper respiratory infection. Two aspirin gave some relief, but that evening he also developed a slight cough, fever of 100 degrees and a general achy feeling. His wife called their family physician, Dr. Levinson, who reviewed the symptoms over the phone. Everything certainly sounded like the classic flu syndrome, which usually gets better in three to seven days. Dr. Levinson reinforced the need for aspirin and asked to be called in two days if there was no improvement.

The next morning Mr. Woodbury was worse. He ached all over and his cough was painful, so he went to see Dr. Levinson, who listened to his heart and lungs and heard nothing unusual. Eyes, ears, nose and throat were normal except for a flushing of the mucous membranes. On the outside chance that this was a bacterial infection, he prescribed an antibiotic, erythromycin, to be taken four times a day. He reassured Mr. Woodbury and asked him to call the next day if he was no better.

That evening Mr. Woodbury developed a mild sensation of shortness of breath, what physicians call dyspnea. Partly for this reason he had a restless night and the next morning, January 13, was back in Dr. Levinson's office. Now there was also a new physical finding, cyanosis, a slight bluish skin color indicating insufficient oxygen in the blood. Dr. Levinson also found Mr. Woodbury's breathing heavier and deeper than normal. Everything pointed to a lung problem, so a chest x-ray was taken immediately. It was not normal. In the right lung was a grapefruit-sized, irregular white shadow just above the diaphragm, consistent with some type of pneumonia. Thirty minutes later Mr.

Woodbury was admitted to the Medical Center's ICU (intensive care unit) with a presumed diagnosis of viral pneumonia.

The pace is fast in the ICU. Within the hour Mr. Woodbury gave a brief history to two doctors and a sputum sample to one of them, had a physical examination, several blood tests, and another chest x-ray, and began receiving intravenous fluids. One of the blood tests, known as arterial blood gas, showed his oxygen pressure dangerously low at 37 millimeters of mercury. Normal PO_2, as the test is abbreviated, is 85 to 100. To help counteract his hypoxia, an oxygen mask was set up to deliver 60% oxygen — almost triple the amount in room air.

I saw Mr. Woodbury soon after admission. His overall appearance can be described as "acutely ill" — an observation based mainly on his dusky skin color, sweat over his brow and obvious breathing difficulty. Also, his muscular build and full, round face made it certain he hadn't been ill for very long. Despite being short-winded he was alert and cooperative. He also seemed strangely optimistic for someone so precipitously admitted to hospital, as if he perceived his condition to be easily curable by medical science. He had no particular reason to be cheerful, so I sensed this was his way of reassuring Mrs. Woodbury, who had just seen him and was now out in the waiting room.

I learned something of their family situation. The Woodburys had two children, ages four and seven. He worked as a foreman at the Ford Motor plant and his wife held a part-time secretarial job in the mornings while their younger child was in day care. Neither his children nor Mrs. Woodbury had been ill recently. Mr. Woodbury had not been hospitalized before, in fact had never been very sick, and did not smoke. He also had not been recently exposed to noxious fumes, chemicals or dusts.

I went to see Mrs. Woodbury, a petite and pretty woman in her mid-30's. She was scared, which considering the circumstances was an appropriate reaction. Before I could explain his problem she wanted to know just how sick he was and "would he make it?" She might have sensed something in my demeanor, or my lack of smile or the way I held my head. (Some ICU physicians believe in laying out all the worst possibilities from the very beginning, at least to the patient's family. This is called "hanging crepe," referring to the black fabric displayed at wakes or funerals. Once this approach is taken, anything bad that happens will have been expected; anything good will make the physician look like a hero. The truth is, I had seen many patients similar to Mr. Woodbury and "guarded" was an optimistic prognosis. Patients with such a rapidly progressive pneumonia can be dead a few days after their first symptoms. Still, except in the most obvious cases of brain anoxia, to emphasize only the worst possibilities is not fair to the family and could even be self-fulfilling.)

I told Mrs. Woodbury that her husband had severe viral or bacterial pneumonia and it was seriously interfering with oxygen delivery into his blood. His course appeared so rapid that if he did not begin to recover soon he would need artificial ventilation and even that would provide only temporary support. We would order specific diagnostic tests, such as blood cultures and microscopic examination of his sputum, and continue treatment with oxygen and antibiotics. He would either respond or not and we would know in 24 to 48 hours. There was a reasonable possibility he would improve but I could give no odds. She accepted this, which is to say all of her immediate questions were answered. I also called Dr. Levinson at his office and told him of the situation. He agreed with our approach.

The initial tests revealed increased numbers of infection-fighting white cells, both in his blood and sputum. We also found his sputum devoid of any bacteria — a finding which could be explained by his already brief use of erythromycin, which might have suppressed their growth. Alternatively, he could be infected with organisms that don't show up on routine sputum examination — this includes all viruses and many bacteria as well. In any case, the chest x-ray, white cell count and sputum exam all suggested a diagnosis of pneumonia, but did not reveal what specific type. Dozens of different organisms — including many species of virus, bacteria, fungi and protozoa — could be responsible.

(By January 1982 AIDS had just been described and most physicians had never seen a case. Therefore AIDS was never suspected in Mr. Woodbury, although we did look for organisms now commonly associated with AIDS infections.)

We started Mr. Woodbury on two intravenous antibiotics, erythromycin and oxacillin. It was decided to continue the erythromycin because that is the best treatment for Legionnaire's disease, which we had not ruled out, and also for mycoplasma pneumonia. The bacteria responsible for mycoplasma pneumonia (*mycoplasma pneumoniae*) and Legionnaire's disease (*legionella pneumophila*) share certain characteristics: both are difficult to diagnose in the first few days of illness; neither can be seen under the microscope using conventional laboratory methods; infections caused by both usually respond to erythromycin. Thus the drug seemed a logical choice for Mr. Woodbury. Oxacillin, a relative of penicillin, was chosen because it is excellent against staphylococcus. Staphylococci are a much more virulent group of bacteria than either *mycoplasma* or *legionella*; whenever a serious "staph" infection is suspected, treatment is begun immediately, without waiting for confirmation.

Mr. Woodbury did not respond. A few hours later he was still dyspneic and cyanotic and his PO_2 was only 45. An oxygen pressure this low — especially while receiving extra oxygen — is always life-threatening. Improving oxygenation at this point would require a major change in management since the oxygen mask was ineffective. Mr. Woodbury needed artificial ventilation, which meant placing a tube in his trachea (the throat), a procedure called endotracheal intubation. We asked the anesthesiologist on call to come up to the ICU and intubate Mr. Woodbury.

Normal breathing, which involves inhaling and exhaling 10 to 16 times a minute, is silent, automatic and effortless. It is also not obvious to the observer. Mr. Woodbury was now breathing 40 times a minute and working very hard at it. From across the room anyone could see his neck muscles rise and fall, a sure sign of increased work of breathing — yet each breath was ineffectual and their sum not enough to sustain life.

Despite severe respiratory distress he remained alert, so I carefully explained what was about to happen. I told him intubation was absolutely necessary (the ventilator could not work otherwise), that he would have to be sedated for the procedure and that even when awake he would not be able to talk or eat.

The artificial ventilator would take over the work of breathing for him. He understood and asked me to call his wife, who had since gone home. I said I would call her afterwards. Fortunately the intubation was quick and successful; he required 10 milligrams of intravenous Valium for sedation.

The ventilator — a machine about the size of a dishwasher — was hooked up to his endotracheal tube via plastic hoses about two inches wide. The dials were set to deliver 14 breaths per minute, with the volume of each breath quadruple the amount he was breathing on his own. To make it easier for him to tolerate the endotracheal tube and not fight the ventilator we gave him another 10 milligrams of Valium.

A chest x-ray was taken with a portable machine; it now showed an abnormal whitish haze in both lungs. (An x-ray film is like the photographic negative of a black-and-white print. A white haze or shadow appears whenever pneumonia or some other abnormality blocks the x-ray beams. Bony structures such as ribs also block the beams and appear white on x-rays. Normal lung, which is mostly thin tissue surrounded by air, lets the x-rays through to develop that part of the film, which then appears black between white ribs.)

At this point the admitting diagnosis seemed correct — viral pneumonia. His sputum revealed no bacteria and it was too early for culture reports to confirm any other diagnosis. But Mr. Woodbury's distress was due to more than just viral pneumonia. In just a few hours once-healthy lung tissue had come apart, allowing plasma to leak out and flood spaces where only air should be . His chest x-ray showed the progression clearly. This acute flooding-known medically as acute pulmonary edema — is not what you see in the usual case of viral (or any other) pneumonia. His problem had progressed beyond simple pulmonary infection.

* * *

Mr. Woodbury now displayed all the classic features of ARDS, the adult respiratory distress syndrome: acute onset of severe respiratory distress; bilateral "white-out" on the chest x-ray; life-threatening hypoxia. ARDS is one of those medical entities that has been around for a long time, but only recently recognized and defined. ARDS was first characterized in a 1967 article published in THE LANCET, England's famous medical weekly. (The authors were all from the University of Colorado Medical Center — it is not unusual for Americans to publish first descriptions of disease in THE LANCET.) Drs. David Ashbaugh, D. Boyd Bigelow, Thomas Petty and Bernard Levine described twelve patients admitted to the Rocky Mountain Regional ICU, all of whom had symptoms and clinical findings similar to each other and to Mr. Woodbury: respiratory distress, severe hypoxia, leakage of fluid into both lungs and a need for artificial ventilation. These symptoms in the twelve patients were precipitated by several different events, including viral pneumonia, pancreatitis and trauma to the chest or abdomen. A few of the patients were in shock prior to the onset of their respiratory distress. ("Shock lung" is sometimes used to mean ARDS; the latter is a much broader term, as shock is only one of many conditions that can precede ARDS.)

Five of the twelve patients died, a percentage which has remained about the same to this day. An autopsy of their lungs were a deep-reddish purple, much heavier and darker than normal, air-filled lungs. This reflected the tremendous inflammation and edema characteristic of ARDS.

ARDS was certainly not new in 1967. The type of patient with severe lung leakage has been described increasingly in the medical literature since World War I, when injured soldiers were often observed to die in fulminant (sudden) respiratory failure. Autopsy studies in the 1930s and 1940s showed that many patients dying of shock had heavy, beefy lungs. In the 1950s and early 1960s severe respiratory distress was described after such disparate conditions as open-heart surgery, compound leg fractures and viral pneumonia. In 1966 the term "DaNang lung" was coined to describe the respiratory complications of soldiers critically wounded in Vietnam. In retrospect most — if not all — of these patients exemplified the adult respiratory distress syndrome.

The importance of the 1967 paper was in recognizing a

pattern of injury not unique to one cause but the final pathway for multiple causes, and in describing the clinical features of ARDS. This subsequently allowed many patients with ARDS to be diagnosed, studied and treated in a rational, uniform fashion.

Precise statistics are unavailable, but when all the causes are considered ARDS turns out to be a common problem. In this country an estimated 75,000 to 100,000 new cases of ARDS occur each year, with about half of the patients surviving. A true incidence is difficult to come by since most ARDS cases end up classified in some other disease category, such as "viral pneumonia" or "multiple trauma." Most ARDS patients are under the age of 65 with no prior history of lung disease. ARDS is not due to heart failure, although a rapidly failing heart can sometimes cause a similar clinical picture. (Some physicians prefer the terms "cardiac pulmonary edema" for severe heart failure and "non-cardiac pulmonary edema" for ARDS.)

ARDS is distinct from infant respiratory distress syndrome, also known as hyaline membrane disease — a condition that claimed the life of John and Jacqueline Kennedy's son on August 9, 1963, two days after birth. Infant ARDS is due solely to premature birth and lack of a normal lung chemical called surfactant. While lack of surfactant plays a role in ARDS, it is not the primary cause.

Little has been learned about the pathophysiology of ARDS since 1967. Basically it involves the leakage of plasma and protein out of pulmonary capillaries, flooding millions of tiny airspaces. (Our lungs are a collection of 300,000,000 or so microscopic airspaces, called alveoli; each alveolus is surrounded by numerous capillaries that take in oxygen and give off carbon dioxide. Normally the barrier between the airspaces and capillaries allows gases to exchange but nothing else, certainly not plasma and large protein molecules.) Why plasma and proteins leak out of the capillaries is not known. There are many theories but none is universally or even widely accepted.

One problem in understanding ARDS is that most patients suffering the commonly-associated medical conditions, such as shock or viral pneumonia, do not end up with leaky lungs. It is for unknown reasons that some victims manifest florid pulmonary edema while others, in a similar clinical situation, maintain fluid-free lungs.

Though there have been some advances in the management of ARDS, none is considered specific therapy; in the jargon of intensive care they are referred to as "supportive," as opposed to "curative." One general advance is the ICU itself, a development dating from the 1930s when polio victims were first concentrated for better care. The modern ICU, with electronic monitoring, artificial ventilators and specially trained staff, evolved in the 1960s and spread nationwide in the 1970s. Today every hospital of more than minuscule size has at least one area where modern monitoring technology and skilled nursing are concentrated. This is the true meaning of intensive care. (Though the concept of the ICU makes a lot of sense intuitively, the benefit of ICUs in reducing mortality has not been proved for most illnesses, including ARDS. Given the critical condition of these patients and the fact that only half may survive the illness, it is not a study anyone cares to perform; no one wants to give any ARDS patient less care than that available in the modern ICU.)

Another advance is the artificial ventilator, which has become more compact and reliable over the years. Unlike the old iron lungs, which hampered nursing contact with the patient's, today's artificial ventilators stand at the side of the bed and are connected to the patient through flexible tubing. They pump air into the lungs, rather than suck air from around the chest cage, which is what the iron lungs did. And modern ventilators can work round the clock for weeks with no more than routine bedside maintenance. It is seldom that any patient dies today from inability to be machine-ventilated.

Today's ventilators are also able, at the twist of a knob, to deliver positive end-expiratory pressure, known worldwide as "PEEP" (pronounced to rhyme with beep). This extra airway pressure-maintained at the end of each breath — helps keep the alveoli open longer so more oxygen can enter the blood. PEEP for ARDS was first reported in the 1967 paper, although its roots go back much further. In the late 1940s pioneering jet aircraft pilots used positive-pressure face masks to increase their oxygen pressure at high altitudes.

Clinical use of PEEP was only conjecture until the Colorado physicians placed five of their ARDS patients on positive airway pressure. Three of the five lived whereas only two of the seven non-PEEPed patients survived. Because of the small numbers of patients these results were, in the parlance of medical investigation, merely anecdotal, but they were enough to place PEEP in the pantheon of ICU techniques. PEEP's main use is to increase oxygen pressure in the blood without using extremely high, and potentially toxic, concentrations of inhaled oxygen.

PEEP is not without hazards; because of the increase in positive airway pressure the lungs can sometimes "blow out" like a burst tire. PEEP can also prevent the normal flow of blood into and out of the heart and cause heart failure. Those complications are manageable — and to a large extent preventable — with careful monitoring.

Machines that easily and rapidly measure blood oxygen and carbon dioxide tensions (the "blood gases") are another evolutionary development. Various methods for blood gas measurement have been available for decades, but technically easy and rapid measurements only since the late 1950s when new types of gas electrodes were introduced. Today, caring for critically-ill patients without blood gas measurements would seem like driving fast in a dense fog. You might make it but you would probably crash. Before the blood gas test was widely available physicians literally guessed at the blood oxygen and carbon dioxide tensions. It was a real crapshoot. Doctors now appreciate the unreliability, for sick patients, of clinically assessing blood gases.

Yet another advance has been a special type of cardiac catheter — a long, thin tube about 1/16 inch wide with a tiny, inflatable balloon on one end. The catheter is trademarked "Swan-Ganz" (Edwards Laboratories, Inc., Santa Ana, California) after H.J.C. Swan and William Ganz, two Los Angeles cardiologists. Drs. Swan and Ganz (along with four others) published their now classic article in a 1970 issue of the NEW ENGLAND JOURNAL OF MEDICINE, "Catheterization of the Heart in Many with use of a Flow-Directed Balloon-Tipped Catheter." Since then "Swan-Ganz" catheterization has taken ICU's by storm. ICU staff speak of inserting a "Swan-Ganz,"

"Swanning" the patient or of the patient being "swanned." No other medical proprietary name has become so universalized in recent memory. (In fact in the early 1990s there is something of a backlash; some physicians feel the catheters are used too freely and when less invasive diagnostic methods would be just as good.)

Most patients who develop ARDS (or one of several other critical heart-lung problems) will sooner or later have a Swan-Ganz catheter placed in their heart. The single major advantage over any previously used catheter is its ability to be accurately placed from the bedside. The patient does not have to be removed to a catheterization lab and, furthermore, bedside measurements can now be obtained on a continuous basis.

(The Swan-Ganz catheter modifies an old technique. Credit for the first cardiac catheterization is given to the German physician Werner Forssmann, whose story is now legend. In 1929, as a recently-graduated doctor working at Augusta-Viktoria Hospital in Eberswalde, near Berlin, Dr. Forssmann conceived the idea of threading a long, thin catheter through an arm vein and into one of the heart's right-sided chambers. His superior refused permission for such a daring study, so Dr. Forssmann clandestinely did it anyway — using himself as subject. He confirmed the catheter's placement with a chest x-ray and published the results in Klinische Wochenschrift later that year. The medical possibilities lay dormant until the 1940s when Dickinson W. Richards, Jr., and Andre Cournand, working at Bellevue Hospital, began a systematic study of heart catheterization. Their work revolutionized cardiac diagnosis and paved the way for open heart surgery. In 1956 Drs. Forssmann, Richards and Cournand shared the Nobel Prize for Physiology or Medicine.)

One of many measurements taken via the Swan-Ganz catheter can tell if a patient has heart failure and serve as a guide to rational fluid management. Patients intubated and artificially ventilated can easily become dehydrated or over-hydrated — normal mechanisms for regulating thirst obviously do not operate. Without these measurements it is often impossible to know how much intravenous fluid to give; the physical examination, chest x-ray and routine lab studies are totally unreliable for this purpose.

Despite these and other advances, and even though we surely manage the syndrome more rationally, have more measurements and understand the physiology much better than a generation ago, the mortality rate in ARDS still hovers around 60%. This was true in 1967, in 1982 (when Mr. Woodbury was care for), and now. Statistics for ARDS mortality before the mid-1960s are not known, mainly because the heterogeneous nature of the syndrome was not recognized. But it is not unreasonable to assume a much higher ARDS mortality without modern intensive care.

The key to treatment is supporting the patient long enough for the lungs to heal. Once lungs fail in their capacity to deliver oxygen either they must recover in a short time or the patient dies. Artificial ventilation for lung failure is measured in days or weeks, not months or years. There is no long-term "dialysis" as exists for kidney failure. If the patient is not destined to recover lung function, no amount of support can keep him alive indefinitely.

Patients who don't recover usually succumb to sepsis, cardiac arrhythmia, internal bleeding or some other catastrophe. One of the saddest spectacles in medicine is to see a patient die with progressive respiratory failure despite the panoply of state-of-the-art, intensive-care technology. Amazingly, those who recover from ARDS, which is surely one of the most serious insults to afflict any organ, end up with normal or nearly normal lung function. ARDS seems to be an all-or-nothing phenomenon.

*   *   *

On the ventilator Mr. Woodbury's PO_2 went up to 84 millimeters of mercury. This was adequate but far from normal, since he was inhaling 80% oxygen — almost four times the normal concentration. An expected PO_2 under these conditions is over 400. He was also receiving PEEP at 10 centimeters of water pressure, a moderate amount.

We gave him two grams of an intravenous corticosteroid, a powerful anti-inflammatory hormone often given empirically for ARDS in the early 1980s (today the drug is used much more sparingly in ARDS patients). Through a neck vein we inserted a

Swan-Ganz catheter and threaded it into his heart. Unfortunately the catheter did not work at first, or rather the measurements did not make sense, as sometimes happens.

A chest x-ray revealed the problem. The catheter tip was coiled inside Mr. Woodbury's chest. After pulling back and reinserting the catheter we were able to get the measurements needed to guide fluid therapy.

This was the scene about 7 p.m., some nine hours after Mr. Woodbury's admission. A young, previously healthy man lay semi-conscious in bed, sedated with Valium. In addition to the endotracheal tube, now firmly taped to his face so as not to slip out, four other tubes violated his body: the Swan-Ganz catheter, through a neck vein; an intravenous catheter, through an arm vein; a special arterial catheter, previously inserted into the radial artery in his right wrist and used for drawing blood gases and monitoring blood pressure; and a soft rubber bladder tube, earlier placed through his penis so that urine output could be measured.

Clear plastic tubing connected the several bags of intravenous fluid to Mr. Woodbury's body; in the aggregate all the tubes looked like vines of some science-fiction forest. Interspersed between the vines were several pieces of electronic monitoring equipment: one to measure heart rate and rhythm, another to display the Swan-Ganz readings and a third to show his blood pressure. Just to the right of his head was the ventilator with its reassuring "whoosh" of air being pumped into his lungs, a sound repeated 14 times every minute.

(At a glance, scenes like that surrounding Mr. Woodbury may appear unreal, certainly not the picture of human care. Doctors and nurses sometimes have to remind themselves that ICU patients like Mr. Woodbury are in fact human, possessing normal capacity to live and love. When we forget this we are dealing not with patients as much as "heart-lung preparations," and the outcome is no more important than an interesting experiment. Intensive care can certainly give the appearance of an exercise in gross physiology. In truth, like some technologic fail-safe mechanism, internal reminders of the patient's humanity constantly arise and help guide us.)

After discussing the next twelve hours' care with the nurses and resident staff left for the evening. Mr. Woodbury was one of five intensive care patients in our ICU at the time, yet by far the sickest. No major changes in therapy were planned and we hoped for an uneventful night.

The next morning, January 14, Mr. Woodbury was not much better. During ICU rounds we reviewed the accumulated data: several chest x-rays, many blood test results, microbiology reports of his sputum, vital sign sheets. We double-checked the medication records and nursing reports. He was receiving the drugs on time and in the correct amount. Throughout the night he had been suctioned frequently and turned in his bed as recommended (lying in one place for prolonged periods is bad for any patient, especially those with ARDS). There was no doubt in anyone's mind — Mr. Woodbury was receiving superb nursing and doctor care, yet he was not improving.

The information so far pointed to an infectious pneumonia as the initial event. Was he on the right antibiotics? The lack of definitive culture reports (still too early for many organisms to grow) and absence of bacteria in his sputum suggested a virus or one of the difficult-to-diagnose bacteria. Could he instead have an unusual fungal or parasitic infection, also difficult to uncover and requiring altogether different antibiotics? And if so, how did he get it? Mr. Woodbury had no history of a compromised immune system, the common setting for "opportunistic infections" (so-called because ordinary fungi and parasites take the opportunity to invade a weakened host). Unusual infections can also occur in bird-handlers, pigeon-breeders and farmers, occupations remote from anything in his experience.

We decided to ask for help and called Dr. Dumont of the Infectious Disease Service. Since Dr. Dumont also ran the microbiology lab he already knew about Mr. Woodbury, at least about all his negative lab results. He sent his clinical fellow to the ICU and an hour later Dr. Dumont himself appeared, fully armed with all the data and his tentative conclusions. He didn't waste any time.

"You've got to treat him for Legionnaire's and pneumocystis." We had continued the erythromycin because of possible Legionnaire's disease and had considered pneumocystis, but thought it a highly unlikely infection in Mr. Woodbury. Pneumocystis is a protozoan that occasionally invades kidney-transplant recipients and immunologically-compromised infants, but rarely healthy adults. Until Mr. Woodbury became suddenly ill, he was a healthy adult.

"I don't think it's pneumocystis but we can't be sure," he continued. "Let's stop the oxacillin and add Bactrim. If he doesn't respond in 48 hours we'll consider an open lung biopsy. Meantime, up his steroids to four grams a day and send a serum sample to the lab for fungal titers."

Bactrim — a trade name for trimethoprium-sulfamethoxasole — is the one of two major drugs for *pneumocystis carinii* pneumonia (the same pneumonia common in AIDS patients). Bactrim is effective and at the same time relatively free of major side effects. Since there was no reason not to follow his recommendations we ordered the Bactrim and increased the steroid dose.

As for open-lung biopsy, this is major surgery and used for diagnosis only as a last resort. There was also no assurance that a piece of Mr. Woodbury's lung, under the microscope, would in fact yield an answer. He was not ready for an open-lung biopsy.

In the afternoon I met with Mrs. Woodbury. She came without the children, mainly because ICU policy does not permit children to visit. I told her about Dr. Dumont and our suppositions. She was not discouraged but also not encouraged. It was just too early to know which way her husband was headed.

Dr. Levinson also came by and we discussed the case. He reassured me that nothing important was missed in Mr. Woodbury's past history and that whatever precipitated this crisis was acute and probably infectious. (Although private family physicians frequently will follow their patients in the ICU, it is not feasible to manage any critically ill patient from an outside office. It's no reflection on primary-care physicians, in this case Dr. Levinson, to have their ICU patients under the care of full time, hospital-based doctors. It is simply the best arrangement for the patient, a fact most office-based physicians well appreciate.)

The rest of the day Mr. Woodbury maintained a PO_2 in the 60s on 10 centimeters of PEEP and 60% oxygen. On the evening of January 14, his second day in the hospital, his PO_2 suddenly dropped to 35; a portable chest x-ray showed that his endotracheal tube had slipped into his right lung, effectively bypassing his left lung which was now collapsed. The tube was pulled back, restoring breathing to both lungs and pushing the PO_2 back up to 59 — still a low level but not life-threatening. A check of his electrocardiogram, urine output and blood pressure uncovered no damage from the transient hypoxia.

On January 15 we received the preliminary culture, microbiology and toxicology reports from specimens taken on admission. (On the outside chance some toxic chemical was the culprit a complete "toxic screen" of his urine and blood had been ordered the day of admission.) Everything so far was negative: there was no obvious or easily-diagnosed bacterial infection or toxin. This did not exclude the possibility of Legionnaire's, *mycoplasma* or a viral infection — all organisms which usually take weeks to diagnose because they require a convalescent blood specimen. (Antibody levels in the convalescent specimen are compared with levels when the patient is acutely ill; a diagnosis is made when antibody to the infecting organism increases four-fold in the interval.)

So forty-eight hours after admission we had no way of knowing what Mr. Woodbury had or if our treatment was effective. Whether or not he would improve seemed as likely to depend on the natural course of his illness as on any treatment. On Dr. Dumont's advice we continued the erythromycin and Bactrim. Throughout January 15 his temperature hovered between 101 and 102 degrees.

There was still no improvement on January 16. His PO_2 ranged between 50 and 60, on 60% oxygen and 10 centimeters of PEEP; the chest x-ray continued to display a "whiteout" in both lungs; and we continued to use small doses of Valium to sedate him and allow the machine to keep him alive. The steroids had not only caused his body to become puffy, a predictable side effect, but had also produced diabetes, a not uncommon result when massive doses are used; his blood sugar went to over 400 milligrams percent (normal is less than 100) and required insulin injections to control.

Now the picture was bleak, not because he was worse but because he was not improving. Patients who don't improve invariably die; ARDS is not a chronic condition anyone can live with. In desperation we began to consider an open-lung biopsy. What would a lung biopsy offer? Not much, unless he had some weird infection we had otherwise missed. What were the risks? General anesthesia and major — albeit technically not difficult — surgery in a critically ill patient. Perhaps an operative mortality rate of one or two percent. We discussed the procedure with his wife, with Dr. Dumont and, tentatively, with the thoracic surgeon. Somewhat reluctantly — since doubted it would be revelatory — we scheduled a lung biopsy for January 18.

He showed the first sign of improvement on January 17. You wouldn't know it unless you had been following his blood gases. He certainly looked no different and his x-ray still showed the diffuse haze in both lungs. But his PO_2 was now up to 95 on the same concentration of oxygen. This indicated some microscopic clearing of his lungs, not yet visible on the x-ray. In retrospect this was a dramatic turnaround.

We lowered his oxygen concentration a little and still his PO_2 held. On 50% oxygen, four hours later, his PO_2 was 92. We left things there. Something was working, probably the natural healing process we had been hoping for. We had no way of knowing if the steroids or antibiotics or PEEP or all three (or none) had helped turn his course. As often happens in ARDS, there was no indication of why he was suddenly improving. We canceled the lung biopsy.

On January 18, breathing 40% oxygen, his PO_2 was 123. The pattern was now one of definite and sustained improvement. Except for the side effects of the steroids and the discomfort of the various tubes, Mr. Woodbury was doing well. We had stopped the sedatives and he was alert. His x-ray also began to show some clearing, the white areas melting away to reveal normal or clear lung fields. We removed the Swan-Ganz and arterial catheters and his urine tube.

As suddenly as he had deteriorated, he got better. Miraculously, we were able to disconnect the ventilator on the afternoon of January 18. The endotracheal tube was left in place another two hours, just in case he became worse, and he received humidified oxygen through the tube. There was no problem and he was able to breathe on his own, through the tube.

About 4 p.m. that afternoon the endotracheal tube was pulled out of his throat.

Followup

Mr. Woodbury was discharged from the ICU on January 20 and from the hospital on January 24. He returned to work February 15. I saw him as an outpatient the following week, at which time breathing tests, including an arterial blood gas, were near normal. Convalescent antibody titers were drawn. At a followup visit in June he was still doing well. Except for some slight decrease in exercise tolerance he has suffered no noticeable aftereffects.

He doesn't remember much of his ICU experience. He does remember going to the hospital and can recall the physical setting in the ICU, but most details, even from a patient's point of view, remain a blur.

We never made a specific diagnosis. All the antibody titers were non-diagnostic. In retrospect, considering all the negative laboratory results, a viral infection seems most likely, both for his early symptoms and the subsequent picture of ARDS. However, so many strains of virus can cause pneumonia that when only one person is infected (as opposed to an epidemic, like influenza), the responsible virus usually goes undetected.

Most viral illnesses are self-limiting and this seemed to fit Mr. Woodbury's course, except that he developed ARDS and became critically ill. With the aid of intensive-care support — particularly artificial ventilation and round-the-clock care by nurses and doctors — he proceeded to get better on his own. Without this support he would surely have died.

9. Too Much Sugar, Too Little History

On morning rounds Peter Mance, one of the interns in MICU, presented a 30 year-old woman admitted with diabetic coma and ketoacidosis the night before. The patient had developed gastroenteritis two days earlier and stopped taking her daily insulin injections.

Dr. Mance had stayed up with his dehydrated, acidotic patient most of the night, balancing her blood glucose and acid levels with the proper amount of insulin and fluids. Before the insulin era she would probably not have survived hospitalization. Now modern medicine — and a conscientious intern — had changed her condition from critical to stable in less than 12 hours.

In diabetes the body's normal supply of insulin is either absent or deficient. Without insulin, a hormone made by the pancreas, glucose cannot enter the cells and be used as energy. Without insulin glucose accumulates 'outside' the cells, in the blood. Depending on the severity of diabetes the blood glucose level may range from normal to over 10 times normal.

Ketoacidosis, the most extreme state of uncontrolled diabetes, results from a sudden and severe lack of insulin; glucose builds up rapidly, to dangerously high levels. To forestall starvation the cells turn to abundant fat as an alternative fuel. Metabolism of fat, less efficient than that of glucose, causes a buildup of harmful acid products called ketoacids — hence the term diabetic ketoacidosis, or DKA. The hallmark of DKA is an excess of acids and glucose in the blood.

DKA patients are very dehydrated because the extra blood glucose spills into the urine along with a large amount of the body's water. Glucose, a type of sugar, is not normally present in urine. 'Tasting the urine' was an early way to diagnose diabetes (*not* a test of modern medicine). The full name of the disease is from an early description in Latin that referred to the urine: diabetes (to pass through) mellitus (honeyed).

*   *   *

Dr. Mance's patient was a 'textbook' case of DKA. Not every MICU patient has to have triple organ failure or present ungodly ethical dilemmas. This patient, at least, presented a straight-forward problem amenable to therapy. She also provided an opportunity to teach some medical history.

We went in to see her, a pleasant Puerto Rican woman named Carlita Gomez. Mrs. Gomez looked and acted normal, which in itself was remarkable. From just her appearance you would not know how sick she was a day earlier.

"How do you feel?" I asked.

"Much better, doctor."

"What happened that you had to come to the hospital? Did you forget to take your insulin?"

"No. Two days ago I began vomiting and was sick to my stomach. I didn't eat so I didn't take my insulin yesterday or the day before."

"Why didn't you come to the hospital right away, when this all started?"

"I thought it would get better, like a stomach virus or something. Yesterday I got much worse and came to the emergency room."

"What made you finally decide to come yesterday?"

"I felt very dizzy and sick. My boyfriend said I looked very bad and he brought me."

"Peter," I said, "can you describe what she looked like on admission?"

"I saw her about twenty minutes after she arrived to the emergency room. She was very somnolent. I had to arouse her to answer questions, but she was lethargic and couldn't give me any information except her name."

"Was she short of breath?"

"Well, she didn't look like an acute asthmatic or anything, but her breathing was rapid and deep."

Rapid and deep, the classic breathing pattern in DKA, is the body's attempt to balance the excess ketoacids by hyperventilation or 'blowing them off.' The other classic symptom, excessive urination, causes great thirst and water ingestion.

"Mrs. Gomez, were you very thirsty before you came to the hospital?"

"Yes, I must have drank twenty glasses of water yesterday and the day before. I couldn't seem to get enough water."

"I bet you went to the bathroom a lot, too."

"Yes."

"Has this ever happened to you before, that you had to come to the hospital for your diabetes?"

"I once came to the emergency room with the flu and they said my blood sugar was high, but I didn't have to stay in the hospital."

"How long have you had diabetes?"

"Since I was twenty-one."

"Have you taken insulin that long, for ten years?"

"Yes."

"Does anybody else in your family have diabetes?"

"My mother, but she just uses [anti-diabetic] pills. She doesn't need insulin."

"Are you married?"

"I was. I'm divorced."

"Any kids?"

"I have two, a boy seven and a girl ten."

"Did you have any problems with the pregnancies?"

"No. They were both heavy babies, though, and the doctors said that was because of my diabetes."

"Who's taking care of the children while you're in the hospital?"

"My mother."

"Do your kids have diabetes?"

"No, not as far as I know. They seem to be fine."

Further history revealed that Mrs. Gomez was followed in our hospital's diabetes clinic, that she was compliant with her insulin therapy, and that she did not suffer from the potential ravages of the disease, such as kidney failure and vascular disease. She supported herself with income from the state's Aid to Dependent Children program and some help from her mother.

We attributed her exacerbation to non-specific gastroenteritis, an inflammation of the stomach and intestines probably caused by a virus. She stopped taking insulin because she couldn't eat, but this only accelerated the vicious cycle leading to high blood sugar and DKA.

I reviewed Dr. Mance's detailed charting of insulin dose and blood test results. In the emergency room Mrs. Gomez's blood glucose was 948 milligrams%, over nine times the normal value of 80 to 100 milligrams%. Her bicarbonate level was only six, about a quarter normal and indicative of severe acidosis (the lower the bicarbonate, the more acid is in the blood). Dr. Mance's meticulous chart showed that both glucose and bicarbonate levels were returning toward normal, a direct result of insulin and fluid therapy.

"Let's see. She's now receiving two units of insulin an hour, right?"

"Right," said Dr. Mance.

"And her blood glucose is down to two hundred forty and bicarbonate up to nineteen?"

"Yes, those are the latest values," he affirmed.

"Well, it looks like she's on her way to complete recovery. You've done a good job, Peter." Turning to Mrs. Gomez, I asked, "How's your stomach? Do you think you can eat now?"

"I feel much better," she said. "I think I'd like to eat something."

"Peter, let's start her on a soft diet, and advance her to regular food if she tolerates that."

I thanked Mrs. Gomez and we stepped outside her room to continue the discussion.

"We should be able to switch her to subcutaneous insulin later today [the method she used at home]. Let's keep her in MICU until she's off the intravenous insulin."

"OK."

I turned to the medical student, Sarah Miles, a bright and energetic woman about five years younger than Mrs. Gomez. "A fairly typical case of DKA, don't you think, Sarah? Have you had a chance to read about her problem?"

"Yes. I read about it last night."

"Good. You worked her up with Dr. Mance, right?"

"Yes." Sarah was on call the night before and had stayed up to help treat Mrs. Gomez.

"What did you read?"

"I read that DKA patients typically present with hyperventilation and stupor, and that reversal is fairly rapid with treatment, which always consists of fluids and insulin."

"That's right. What did doctors do with these patients before insulin was available? Anybody know?"

There was no answer.

"Starvation," I said. "Doctors prescribed starvation diets to their diabetic patients. Unfortunately, without insulin, almost everyone with ketoacidosis died. How long has insulin been available? Did your book mention that bit of history, Sarah?"

"No, I didn't see that," she replied.

"Well, how old are you, if you don't mind my asking?"

"Twenty-four."

"Was insulin around when you were born, in nineteen sixty-five?"

"I think so," she said, perhaps wondering what the question had to do with our patient.

"Well, was insulin around in nineteen *fifty-five*?"

Bill Sedgwick, the other intern on rounds, spoke up. "I think that's when insulin was introduced. Nineteen fifty-five." He spoke with assurance, as if he really knew the answer.

"Bill," I said in a congratulatory tone, "do you play Trivial Pursuit?"

"Sometimes," he said.

"Anybody disagree with Bill?" I asked. No one answered. Everyone seemed to agree 1955 was when insulin became available. If so, they were only off by three decades.

Ignorance about this seminal event in medicine wasn't their fault, if it could even be called a fault. 'History of medicine' is almost never taught in medical school. Even the historical aspects of everyday diagnosis and therapy are usually omitted. One principal reason is that the teachers are themselves often ignorant or uninterested, and that's too bad.

Doctors interested in history know that it helps provide perspective and humility in daily practice. It teaches us that today's "correct" therapy may be viewed as wrong-headed nonsense by future generations, much as we view primitive therapy of the 19th century and earlier.

Knowledge of historical events can also be of practical importance. For example, anti-tuberculous drug therapy was only introduced in the late 1940s. Anyone who contracted TB before then could not possibly have received effective drug therapy, yet on more than one occasion I've been told on rounds, by some well-meaning medical resident, that a patient received "TB drugs" in the 1930s or early 1940s.

Another time a house officer related a patient's treatment for Legionnaire's disease to a year before the disease was first described (1976)! Even local history is important. A patient could not have had a CAT scan before the machine was available (in our hospital, 1978), yet I have been presented with the results of such phantom scans.

Like any history, of course, medicine's is far more than dates. The pioneering work of Banting, Best, Macleod and Collip in insulin, of Koch in tuberculosis, of Pasteur in rabies, and of Enders and Salk in polio vaccine, cannot be taught by dates alone. The stories behind major medical breakthroughs are invariably full of scientific excitement and human drama (and are well-told in numerous books, such as Paul DeKruif's *Microbe Hunters*, Michael Bliss's *The Discovery of Insulin* and James Watson's *The Double Helix*). Still, it would be helpful if young physicians knew a few important dates.

"Nineteen twenty-two," I said. "Insulin was introduced into clinical medicine in nineteen twenty-two."

"Oh well," said Bill Sedgwick, suggesting by his tone that it really didn't matter whether it was 1922 or 1955.

"The first patient to receive insulin was a thirteen-year-old diabetic boy named Leonard Thompson. In what city?"

If they didn't know the date they also would not know the location of this medical milestone, but I was having fun and they didn't seem to mind.

"Boston," guessed Dr. Sedgwick.

"No."

"New York," said Dr. Miles.

"London?" said one of the nurses, in a final desperate stab.

"No. Everyone give up?"

All did.

"Toronto. The Toronto General Hospital. January eleventh, nineteen twenty-two. And who received a Nobel Prize for the discovery of insulin?"

"Banting," said Dr. Sedgwick, who was still out to win the trivia prize.

"You're half right," I said. "Banting who?"

"That's his last name. I don't remember his first name."

"Did anybody else get the Nobel Prize for work on insulin?"

No answer.

"How about Best? Banting and Best, does that ring a bell?" The two names, of course, are forever linked with the discovery of insulin. Even many grade school students have heard of Banting and Best.

"That's right," said Dr. Sedgwick. "Banting and Best. I remember now."

"Yes," said Dr. Mance. "I remember too. Banting and Best, but I don't remember their first names or anything about them."

"Actually, they are names you probably heard before you entered medical school. Like Salk and Sabin. Probably because of the Nobel Prize, I bet. Salk and Sabin got the Nobel Prize for the polio vaccine, and Banting and Best got it for insulin. Right?"

There was general murmur of agreement.

"Does anyone disagree?" If my questions seemed obnoxious no one complained. In any case I felt compelled to continue, especially since no one disagreed with my purposely erroneous statement about Salk, Sabin, and Best.

"Well, for starters, Sabin and Salk did *not* win the Nobel Prize."

"No? Sure they did," said Dr. Sedgwick. "That can't be."

"Sure they *didn't*. They developed and introduced the polio vaccines, but never got a Nobel Prize for their work. The Prize was given for earlier work on culturing the polio virus in monkey kidney cells, work that was published in 1949. So who got the Prize for work on polio?"

Now they were baffled. I was asking a bit of trivia they must have missed in school. No one answered so I continued.

"The Nobel Prize was awarded to three Americans, Drs. Enders, Robbins, and Weller, in nineteen fifty-four, before the polio vaccine was even released. They were the ones who developed a method to culture the polio virus. Without their work there would have been no vaccine."

"Really?"

"Really. And it was in Boston, too."

"Are you sure Salk and Sabin never got the Nobel Prize?" asked Dr. Sedgwick, still unbelieving.

"I'm sure. They got just about every other prize, but not the one from Stockholm.

"What about Banting and Best? Didn't they get it for discovering insulin?"

"Yes and no. That's an interesting story," I said. "Anybody want to hear it?"

I wasn't sure anyone did, but I wanted to tell it. It is one of the more fascinating stories of medical discovery.

"Yes," said one of the nurses. "Tell us."

"Right," agreed Dr. Mance.

Sensing a trace of sarcasm, I suddenly felt a need to defend the subject of medical history. Looking toward the patient I said, "There's more to a case like this than just glucose and bicarbonate levels. Sometimes we take these modern miracles too much for granted. Since you insist, I'll tell you about the discovery of insulin." And I did.

*   *   *

Before 1922 young diabetics were treated with low-carbohydrate, starvation diets. Even so, patients with DKA invariably died in coma. William Osler, in his 1892 *The Principles and Practice of Medicine*, a standard text of the era, wrote:

> In children the disease [diabetes] is rapidly progressive, and may prove fatal in a few days...as a general rule, the older the patient at the time of onset the slower the course...In

> true diabetes instances of cure are rare...Our injunctions today are those of Sydenham [an earlier physician]: 'Let the patient eat food of easy digestion, such as veal, mutton, and the like, and abstain from all sorts of fruit and garden stuff.' The carbohydrates in the food should be reduced to a minimum.

Reflecting medical practice of the day, Osler's text devotes almost a full page to specific dietary recommendations, listing those items which the diabetic may take and those which were prohibited. Among the latter was "ordinary bread of all sorts."

Osler's comment on 'Medicinal treatment' of diabetes was an understatement:

> This is most unsatisfactory, and no one drug appears to have a directly curative influence.

In fact, no drug was even indirectly curative. On the subject of diabetic coma, Osler wrote:

> The *coma* is an almost hopeless complication.

Frederick Banting was a 30-year-old surgeon from London, Ontario who had the idea of isolating the specific secretion of the pancreas that lowers glucose in the blood. By the end of World War I scientists knew some substance in the pancreas acted to lower glucose, but no one had been able to isolate it or use pancreatic extract successfully in diabetic patients. Banting moved to Toronto in 1921 to work in the lab of Dr. John Macleod, a Scottish physiologist who was an expert in the field of carbohydrate metabolism.

Banting was aided in his work by Charles Best, a 22-year-old medical student. The two of them succeeded in preparing an extract of pancreas that did lower blood sugar in dogs. This extract, of course, contained insulin. Under their direction the first human trial of insulin took place in January 1922 (history records earlier animal trials of crude pancreatic extract, most notably by a Georg Ludwig Zuelzer in Berlin, but nothing came of that research).

Leonard Thompson weighed only 64 pounds when he was admitted to Toronto General in December, 1921. His diagnosis: diabetic ketoacidosis. He was initially given a diet consisting of only vegetables [see 'A Case of Diabetes Mellitus', New England Journal of Medicine, February 11, 1982]. Before he received insulin Thompson's blood sugar ranged from 350 to 560 milligrams%.

Thompson was still in the hospital when Banting and Best were ready with their extract in January 1922, so he was the first human to receive it. According to the hospital record, Thompson's blood sugar fell from 470 to 320 milligrams% six hours after the injection.

It took Banting and Best two weeks to get more of the extract and Thompson didn't receive his next injection until January 23. His blood sugar responded by falling each time. Thompson continued to receive insulin and was sent home on May 15, 1922, weighing 67 pounds.

Almost from the very beginning the discovery of insulin sparked controversy. Up until early 1922 Macleod had played no direct role in the discovery. Although he had acted as advisor on a number of the experiments, and Banting and Best used his lab, Macleod was actually out of the country in the summer of 1921 when most of the important dog experiments were accomplished.

The earliest scientific reports listed only Banting and Best as authors. In fact, Banting later wrote that he was discouraged in his work by Macleod, and that Macleod told him that "negative results would be of great physiological value." When it became clear that an important discovery had been made Macleod got involved and orchestrated the production of insulin and further research into its use.

At the time insulin was considered a cure for diabetes so the discovery was quite a sensation. And no wonder. Patients near death were miraculously resurrected after only a few injections of the vital hormone. As expected, the discovery lead to the Nobel Prize for Physiology or Medicine. It was awarded in the fall of 1923 to Banting and . . . Macleod.

Upon hearing of the award Banting was furious. In his view, Macleod had done none of the original work but only impeded his own brilliant research. Banting thought Charles Best should have shared the Prize.

Since Best was only a student at the time, and did not present any of the research at meetings, as did Banting and Macleod, his role in the discovery was not prominently featured. The Nobel committee was aware of Best (he was co-author on the original papers) but was more impressed by Macleod's senior status and the fact that he presented much of the research at scientific gatherings, one of which was attended by a Nobel committeeman. Also, by intention the Nobel committee wanted to honor only two recipients (it was not until 1945 that three people would share a Nobel Prize in Physiology or Medicine). To the Nobel committee in Sweden Banting and Macleod seemed the logical choices.

Banting tried to correct the injustice by giving half of his award to Best (the total monetary award in 1922 was $24,000). As it turns out another scientist was also overlooked by the Nobel committee, a biochemist named J.D. Collip. Collip was responsible for purifying insulin far beyond what Banting and Best had achieved with their crude extract. In fact Collip had purified all the injections given the Thompson boy except the first one. After being apprised of Banting's gesture Macleod shared half of *his* prize money with Collip.

For the next two decades there was bitter (and private) feuding among all four men over priorities and who did what. Banting continued to believe that Macleod had hogged the limelight and deserved no credit for the discovery of insulin. Macleod thought Banting was an ungrateful young doctor who didn't appreciate how much he, the senior professor, had contributed to the discovery. Best, of course, was truly slighted by the Nobel Committee and many contemporaries felt he should have been named a recipient of the Prize.

At least Best's contribution has been fully recognized by history, not to mention the University of Toronto. He outlived everyone in the story, dying in 1978 after a distinguished career as a professor of physiology. Collip also achieved long-lasting recognition for his pioneering work on purifying insulin. Macleod died in 1935, in Scotland. As for Banting, he died in a plane crash in Newfoundland in 1941.

*   *   *

"Well, that's enough about the discovery of insulin," I said. "Anybody have any questions?"

"What happened to the boy who got the insulin?" asked Dr. Sedgwick.

"Oh, glad you asked that. He lived another thirteen years, dying in nineteen-thirty-five at age twenty-seven, of severe bronchopneumonia. They did an autopsy and found the ravages of diabetes, including a shrunken pancreas."

"Any more questions?" There were none.

"OK," I said, "let's go see the next patient."

10. Crusade

Harlan Tembo, 57, has chronic bronchitis, a result of smoking cigarettes since he was 15. Mr. Tembo was brought to Memorial Medical Center's emergency room one Monday in respiratory distress, blue, semi-conscious, and about to die. His diagnosis: severe bronchitis and acute respiratory failure. He was intubated, connected to a ventilator and sent to MICU.

His hospital care reflected a quiet revolution in medicine. Before ventilators were available for patients like Mr. Tembo — that is, before the 1960s — he would have died. Today patients with acute and otherwise fatal lung failure are often saved by just a few days of 'ventilator support.' Even chronic patients with end-stage lung disease can benefit if their respiratory failure is acute and reversible. One of Memorial's chronic lung disease patients has been intubated at least nine times for acute respiratory failure. For Mr. Tembo, it was his first time intubated.

As late as 1967 there was debate about the utility of artificial ventilation in respiratory failure. Back then ventilators were much scarcer; now they are commonplace in every hospital. The only real debate over ventilator use today involves ethical issues, not medical ones.

After four days of artificial ventilation Mr. Tembo could breathe on his own, unassisted by machine. It was time to begin my no-smoking crusade.

Every physician should mount a crusade when patients are most vulnerable, which is usually when they are ill and especially when hospitalized. It is not wrong to choose this time; it is wrong not to.

I am amazed how often physicians treat serious illness related to alcohol or tobacco, and do little (or nothing) to educate the patient. Why? Do doctors think patients automatically make the connection between habit and illness? In fact patients all too often fail to make any connection unless directly and specifically told what it is.

Cynics may say I am wasting my time but evidence from various studies suggests otherwise. There is a positive influence on individual patients when *their* doctor gives advice in a forceful and direct manner. This is especially true about smoking.

The advice has to be more than mouthing a few words. The doctor (or nurse, for that matter) has to demonstrate genuine concern for the patient. Sometimes simple repetition will do it. Occasionally a threat works, as in: 'You'll need to find another doctor if you don't quit smoking.'

But how do you communicate to someone you may never see again, or someone with only a grade school education, or someone who is a borderline psychotic? Sometimes reason, logic, and common sense are not enough. The message must always be personal and tailored to the patient's level of understanding. The important thing is to try.

*   *   *

"Let's extubate him," I said.

"Do you think he's ready?" asked one of the interns.

"Sure. He's awake, he's writing notes, he wants the tube out. Right Mr. Tembo?" He gave a vigorous nod. The nurse went to get the few items needed for extubation.

"You know you can never smoke again, Mr. Tembo. We found cigarette smoke in your blood and that's why you ended up in intensive care." He nodded again, as if agreeing just so I wouldn't leave the tube in.

"Once we get this tube out, if you go back to smoking the tube will have to go right back in." Now he shook his head, meaning he wasn't going to smoke again.

The nurse returned with scissors and an oxygen face mask. I cut the tape securing the tube to his face, deflated the cuff inside his throat and pulled the tube out. Extubation is always a pleasure for patients, providing they are not gasping for air in the first place (as was Mr. Tembo on admission). If you can imagine a foot long plastic tube stuck in your throat, making it impossible to speak or swallow or move your mouth, you can imagine the relief when it comes out.

"How do you feel, Mr. Tembo?"

"Better." His voice was hoarse but understandable.

"Do you know where you are?"

"In the hospital."

"When did you come in?"

"Last night."

"What day is it?"

"Tuesday?"

He had lost track of time, not uncommon in patients who receive artificial ventilation for more than a day.

"No. It's Thursday. You came in on Monday. You've been here for four days already. Do you know why?"

"No."

"Your lungs stopped working."

"Really? I guess I'm lucky to be here. Can I eat something?"

"Not right away. We'll let you have a little water, and then some soup." It's best not to give solid food right after a patient has just come off the ventilator.

"I'll be back later to talk to you about that cigarette smoke in your blood." Having finished our immediate task we went to see the rest of our patients.

The next morning Mr. Tembo was like a new man. He had eaten his first regular meal and was well enough to leave MICU.

"Well," I said. "You're much better. You know you were quite sick a few days ago. A machine had to take over your breathing for four days."

"That's what they tell me."

"Do you know why?"

"Bronchitis, I guess."

"Well, that's true. You almost *died*. You came this close to being completely dead." I held up my forefinger and thumb an inch apart. "Do you know how you got that way?"

"No." He really didn't know or understand. But, sensing that the preacher was about to strike and remembering the conversation from the day before, he answered, "Cigarettes?"

"That's right. You almost died from cigarettes. Your blood was filled up with cigarette smoke." (Actually, his blood showed an excess of carbon monoxide, one of the toxic components of cigarette smoke).

"Well, I'm not going to smoke again."

I acted skeptical. "I've heard that before. Should we save this bed for you just in case?"

"Naw, you can give it to someone else. You won't see me back."

Time to stop badgering? Believe him? No. The physician has to make some *impression* on the patient, even to the point of looking silly or sounding obnoxious. Besides, I rationalized, I'm not only communicating with Mr. Tembo, I'm also teaching housestaff. Teaching them what? That they must do more than offer perfunctory advice about smoking.

"Mr. Tembo, I'm afraid your next cigarette could be your last." Then I delivered a non-sequitur: "Do you live near a funeral home?"

"Yes, why?"

"After you get home and decide to start smoking again, go there before you light up. That way, if you die right away they won't have to bring your body to the hospital." (Actually this is not true. Even if you drop dead in the lobby of a morgue, the police will come and remove your body to the closest hospital to be pronounced. After this was pointed out to me I changed 'funeral home' to 'emergency room.')

"Well I'm not going to smoke again, you can bet on that."

"I hope not. But we'll keep a bed open just in case."

Mr. Tembo was discharged after a week in the hospital. He was admitted a year later for another exacerbation of chronic lung disease, but not as bad as the episode recounted above. He did not require intubation or care in MICU. And his blood carbon monoxide level was normal. He had not resumed smoking. "Why not?" I asked him. "Well," he said, "I remember what you told me last year. So I just gave it up. I don't miss it at all."

*   *   *

I don't know how many times I've taken cigarette packs from a patient's bed stand (always with their permission) or used my funeral home (emergency room) plea to get the message across.

Probably a hundred times over the years. If it worked only once it was worth it.

For Amanda Wiggins though, none of my usual messages got through. She has chronic lung disease and always complains of being 'short winded.' That was her constant complaint during one hospitalization on the medical ward (on that occasion she did not need artificial ventilation or care in MICU. Neither fear of funeral homes nor emergency rooms nor ventilators nor lung cancer nor skin wrinkles made any dent in Mrs. Wiggins' smoking addiction. She was incorrigible. She continued to smoke in her hospital room and in the ward lounge even as we treated her for smoking-related lung disease. (This was before our hospital became a smoke-free institution).

Psychiatrically she was a "borderline" personality disorder — not psychotic, but with a tendency in that direction. Her anchor in life seemed to be the bible and fundamentalist religion. I saw this belief as a wedge to change her behavior.

One day on the ward, as she complained about her dyspnea, I auditioned my new message. I made sure her nurse was there; no one would probably believe me if Mrs. Wiggins really did quit smoking.

"Amanda, we can't get you better if you continue to smoke."

"I'll quit," she said, in a manner which conveyed she had no intention of quitting.

"You've got to quit."

"I'll quit. I want to get better."

"You're gonna die!"

"Don't say that, Dr. Martin. If I quit will I get better?"

"How are you going to quit? You've promised me a hundred times and you always go back to smoking."

"Well, I'll quit now."

"Can I have your cigarettes?" I knew her supply was endless; taking them would be like trying to cut off the flow of cocaine with a single arrest. Still, it was a step in the right direction.

"Take 'em," she said confidently. I opened her drawer and took out two unopened packs of cigarettes.

"Can I have the others?"

"I don't have any more. That's all I have," she said.

I knew this woman. She was not about to quit smoking so easily.

"Now you've got to swear you'll quit smoking."

"I'll swear." She said this with no emotion.

"Then swear."

"I swear." Still no emotion. I reached over and picked up her bible.

"Swear on this," I commanded.

"Why do I have to swear on the bible?" Now her voice was rising. "I *said* I wouldn't smoke."

I knew it. She had no intention of quitting. Unless I could get her to swear on the bible she would never take the oath seriously.

"You've got to swear on the bible. Otherwise God won't believe you're sincere."

She hesitated and her body began to shake. She looked at me, then the bible, then at me again.

"Dr. Martin," she said indignantly, her voice now trembling a little, "that's the word of the Lord! You want me to swear on the Bible?"

"Swear!" I was becoming transformed into a medical evangelist. "SWEAR!"

"I can't do that!"

"Then you don't intend to quit."

"But I will quit. I promise!"

"Then SWEAR!"

Slowly, hesitatingly, she placed her right hand on the bible. I felt the adrenalin flow. I was about to make my first convert.

"Repeat after me. I, Amanda Wiggins..."

"I, Amanda Wiggins..."

"Do swear before God in Heaven..."

"Do swear before God in Heaven..."

"That I will never touch or smoke cigarettes again."

"Oh Dr. Martin!"

I repeated the commandment with raised voice. "THAT I WILL NEVER TOUCH OR SMOKE CIGARETTES AGAIN."

"That I will never touch or smoke cigarettes again," she echoed.

"SO HELP ME GOD!" I bellowed.

"So help me God," she responded. With the last word her whole body shook and she began crying. I checked her pulse and listened to her lungs. No acute problem. She was not having an asthma attack, just a religious experience. Had I reached her? I left Ms. Wiggins sobbing quietly on the bed. The nurse watching the scene promised to check her every half hour.
Feeling quite smug about my effort, I went to see other patients. I remember thinking: all it takes to get a patient to quit smoking is to communicate on their level, to search out that part of their psyche that listens to the doctor. Why aren't all physicians this creative with health advice?

A half hour later the nurse called me to come to the ward lounge. "You won't believe this," she said. The tone in her voice punctured my balloon. 'Oh yes I will,' I thought. There in the lounge sat Ms. Wiggins, smoking a cigarette; she looked up at me with not the least hint of anxiety.

"What happened?" I asked, feigning a hurt incredulity. "You PROMISED me you would quit. You promised GOD!"

"I just had to have a cigarette," she said with an innocent smile.

That was the first and last time I tried religion to break a patient's habit.

Comment

In 1964, when the first surgeon general's report on Smoking and Health was published, 40% of adult Americans smoked regularly. Today the figure is 25%, or about 50 million people.

Of the millions who have quit smoking in the past generation, an estimated 90% did so 'cold turkey,' without the aid of any therapy or drugs or behavior modification. Although nicotine in cigarettes can be addicting, once the mental decision is made to quit it is not all that difficult.

Still, for some people like Mrs. Wiggins and the patient in the next story, quitting is out of the question.

11. "Just give me a cigarette!"

Harold Switek has two major diseases — emphysema and paranoid schizophrenia. His lung disease comes from smoking two packs a day for 35 years. Cigarettes did not cause his psychosis, of course. Though "tobaccoism" is a recognized form of addiction mental illness is not a known complication.

Smoking is distressingly common among psychiatric inpatients. It helps to allay their anxiety and attempts to withhold tobacco tend to make things worse. It is almost impossible to get a psychotic patient to quit smoking (schizophrenia is one type of psychosis) and most psychiatrists are reluctant to badger such patients about the harmful effects of tobacco. As a result, although inpatients are forbidden to keep matches smoking is not generally discouraged by a hospital's psychiatry staff. To allow smoking but not matches, many psychiatry wards install a permanent cigarette lighter at the nurse's station.

I knew Mr. Switek's case would be difficult the moment I heard from Dr. Janis, his psychiatrist.

"Larry? Hi. This is Nancy Janis. How are you? Good. I wonder if you could do me a favor."

"Sure Nancy, what is it?"

"I have a 50-year-old man in Weathergill [Psychiatric Pavilion] who's been there two weeks. He's developed a breathing problem and I can't keep him there any longer. They have no medical ward and I'm afraid he needs to be transferred. Would you be able to take him on MICU?"

"Sure. How bad is he? Does he need a ventilator?"

"I don't think so. He has chronic emphysema and we have him on oral meds but he's getting worse. We can't give IV therapy at Weathergill."

"What medication is he taking? Anything that might suppress his breathing?"

"He's had schizophrenia for decades. Poor Harold. He's been in and out of hospitals. I've only had him as a patient the past year. The only thing I can control him with is Thorazine. He's up to 800 milligrams a day but I think that's a safe dose. He might be able to go without it for a while, but he'll eventually need it."

"Oh," I said. "Well, we'll see what he's like. That much Thorazine probably can suppress breathing in someone with severe lung disease. I may have to stop it for a short time."

"What's happening is his emphysema is getting worse. I think he needs IV therapy."

"No problem. When will he arrive?"

"I'll call an ambulance now. He should be there within an hour. I'll make sure they send a copy of his medical records with him."

"What's the situation with relatives? Is he married?"

"No. He lives with his 80-year-old mother. She's all he has. I'll call and let her know."

"OK. We'll call you back if we have questions about his psychiatric management."

"Good. I'll stop by tomorrow and see him anyway."

*   *   *

Mr. Switek arrived on schedule. Since everything was prearranged he came right up to MICU, bypassing the emergency room. My first impression was that he didn't look all that bad. My second impression was that he didn't look all that crazy. I was wrong on both counts.

The MICU nurses put him in bed, took his vital signs, and began setting up an intravenous line. I went in with the intern, Dr. Solomon, to begin our examination. Wearing only shorts and a hospital gown open in the front, he appeared short and stocky, with large thighs and arms. His barrel chest was covered with hair and his abdomen protruded with about 25 excess pounds. The transfer record listed him at 185 pounds, 5 feet 7 inches.

His face was big and round, with a crew cut on top, a feature I've always found incongruous in a middle-aged-man. Although he did not look short of breath one can be fooled by patients at rest, especially those with chronic lung disease. I have seen patients comfortable in bed who could not walk across the room without gasping for air.

On closer observation his breathing problem was more apparent. Dusky skin and lips signified oxygen deficiency, all the more remarkable because he was receiving oxygen through a nasal cannula. Rapid respiratory rate (34 breaths a minute) and contracting neck muscles signified his dyspnea. His blood pressure was normal, heart rate increased, and temperature up slightly to 100 degrees.

Probably because of his psychiatric history I was also cognizant of some subtle features. His eyes were open wider than normal and he gazed through rather than at you. He did not make eye contact for more than a fraction of a second. Also, his speech was rapid, much faster than most patients with severe lung disease.

"Hello, I'm Dr. Martin and this is Dr. Solomon. How are you?"

"I want to call my mother. Is she here? What's your name? What are you going to do? Is my mother here? Where are my shoes? Why can't I have my shoes?"

"She's been called. She knows you're here," I answered calmly. "And you won't need your shoes while you're in MICU."

"She wants me home. I want to go home. Where are my shoes? Hey, can I have a cigarette? Where are my cigarettes?" With his last question he began turning his head from side to side and up to the ceiling, as if we were keeping his cigarettes close by, somewhere in the ICU cubicle.

"You can't go home now, Mr. Switek. You were sent here because of your breathing."

"Hey Doc, there's nothing wrong with my breathing. I just want a cigarette. Can I have a cigarette? Where are my cigarettes? I'll just take one."

"That's impossible, Mr. Switek. You're in the intensive care unit! There's oxygen all around you."

"I'll go outside. Can I have a cigarette?"

"Can I listen to your lungs?"

"OK."

Dr. Solomon and I went right to his lungs and heart, bypassing areas customarily examined first: no telling when he might decide not to cooperate. Facing each other behind Mr. Switek's hairy back, we each placed a stethoscope up and down his chest, listening to him breathe. Our eyes met as our ears heard the same thing: diffuse and severe wheezing, sometimes described as "tight breathing" because it signifies air squeezing through constricted passages.

"Better get a blood gas," I said to Dr. Solomon. He went to get a syringe for the arterial blood sample. I came around the side of the bed to face Mr. Switek.

"Now can I have a cigarette?" he asked, as soon as he saw me.

"You can't smoke!" I gesticulated, flapping my hands up and down for effect. "You'll blow up if you smoke!" (Not true, but I thought this would get to him.)

"Naaah," he said, without missing a beat. "I won't blow up. You're just saying that. Please get me my cigarettes. Where are they?"

"First let's see what our tests show," I said.

"OK. But I can have a cigarette first?"

MICU could handle any type of lung problem. Could we handle a psychotic patient with a lung problem?

Thirty minutes later we had results of arterial blood gas analysis, chest x-ray, and electrocardiogram. Mr. Switek's oxygen level was dangerously low, only 48. The cardiogram showed a heart strain from the low oxygen, and his cardiac rhythm showed skipped beats and other ominous irregularities. Fortunately his chest x-ray was clear — no pneumonia.

Our diagnosis was acute bronchial infection on top of emphysema, with impending respiratory failure. He was almost at the point of needing intubation and artificial ventilation. Perhaps with an increase in inhaled oxygen, plus antibiotics, steroids and other medication, he could get by without intubation.

I went in to tell him the news, realizing he probably wouldn't hear a thing I had to say.

"We have the results of the tests, Mr. Switek. Your lungs are really bad. We're starting treatment with some powerful drugs.

If they work you'll recover from this breathing attack. If not, we might have to sedate you out and put a tube in your throat. Under no circumstances can you smoke. Do you understand?"

"OK. When can I get my cigarettes?"

He was incapable of understanding. It was like talking to a child.

"Look, I'll make a deal with you. Let us treat you for a few days. When you get better you can have a cigarette." Never before had I made such a deal.

"OK," he said.

We discontinued Thorazine since the drug was probably depressing his respiratory drive, and provided supplemental oxygen through a nasal cannula. At this point improving his breathing had a higher priority than treating his psychosis.

Over the next 24 hours his blood oxygen level came up a little but his heart beat still danced around the monitor and his wheezing was as tight as before. We vacillated about whether to intubate him and begin artificial ventilation. There are no numbers to go by for such an important decision, only careful bedside observation coupled with the results from arterial blood gases.

During his first 24 hours in MICU Mr. Switek's breathing became so labored that he actually ceased asking for cigarettes. In the middle of the second day his agitation increased, a probable result of not receiving Thorazine. At Dr. Janis's suggestion we restarted the drug at a much lower dose than she had used before, only 100 milligrams twice a day.

On the evening of the second day Mr. Switek deteriorated rapidly. His breathing became more labored, nostrils flared with each breath, and he looked like a fish out of water. Coupled with cardiac irregularities and poor oxygenation, all signs pointed to the need for artificial ventilation. We called anesthesiology.

The anesthesiologist came and injected him with a quick-acting paralyzing agent; without complete paralysis Mr. Switek would have been too difficult to intubate. Once intubated, the ventilator took over his breathing. We then placed an arterial catheter was placed in his arm so frequent blood samples could be obtained for oxygen and carbon dioxide measurements.

Over the next few hours the ventilator corrected his oxygen and carbon dioxide levels. As the paralysis wore off we began sedative medication so he would sleep; he had not had much sleep since arriving to MICU. We held Thorazine since he was kept under sedation.

With sleep, adequate oxygenation, and antibiotics Mr. Switek's pulmonary condition improved. After two days of artificial ventilation his lungs sounded clear. We stopped the sedation and tested his lung function with the ventilator temporarily disconnected: it was much better. On the morning of his fourth hospital day we pulled the tube out of his throat.

For the next eight hours Mr. Switek was docile: no complaints, no agitation. Then, towards the evening he asked his nurse for a cigarette. She explained that he couldn't smoke.

"Just give me a cigarette," he insisted.

"Harold, you know you can't smoke. You just came off the ventilator," she reasoned.

He did not argue the point. Instead, he waited for her to leave the room. Then he got out of bed to go search for tobacco. This was not so easy in his condition. Mr. Switek had been in bed for four days, two of them unconscious, narcotized. Anyone in his state should get out of bed slowly and always with assistance.

Incredibly, standing up for the first time in several days didn't phase him. He didn't faint or even wobble. However, he still had an arterial catheter in one arm, connected to a monitor, and a venous catheter in the other arm, through which he received antibiotics. As he moved away from the bed each catheter disconnected from its extension tubing. The venous tube dripped dark red blood. The arterial catheter, being in a high pressure vessel, spurted blood of a brighter hue.

"Harold, where are you going?" his nurse called out. Harold didn't answer.

"You'll bleed to death," she exclaimed. This was not an idle threat, as arterial blood continued to spurt from the catheter still in his arm.

"Naaah. I'll be OK. I need a cigarette." He continued walking toward the MICU doors.

The nurse quickly realized he was not about to get back in

bed.

"Let me pull those tubes out of you," she said bravely. He let her. That done, he felt free to roam. Although blood still oozed from the puncture sites at least he would not exsanguinate.

"I want a cigarette," he said to the night clerk at the nurses' station. She got up and walked away.

Two nurses implored him to get back to bed. "OK. Give me a cigarette, OK?"

"We can't, Harold," they pleaded. "Please get back into bed."

He moved on, a sight to behold, walking around the MICU nurses' station wearing only a hospital night shirt and no underwear, with drops of blood dripping to the floor from each arm. Our schizophrenic patient was unconcerned with his appearance or health or the scene he was causing. He was possessed with a single idea — CIGARETTE! The nurses kept their distance. One of them called Security. Then me.

Meanwhile, Mr. Switek found his way to the swinging doors that separate MICU from the waiting area. No one tried to stop him. He walked out the doors and down the hallway toward the elevators, where he was met by the security team of two large men.

"Where are you going?"

"I'm looking for a cigarette machine." (There is none in the hospital).

"You have to get back to your room, Mr. Switek." He asked them for a cigarette. They proceeded to escort him back to MICU. He may have thought they were taking him to a cigarette machine, as he did not offer any resistance.

I arrived in MICU just as he was being escorted back by the officers. At the entrance to his room it dawned on him that he wasn't being lead to a cigarette machine and he turned around rapidly to go the other way.

At this point the scene became physical. He had to be restrained to prevent injury to himself (he would have walked in front of a moving car to get a cigarette). The two guards with the help of a male nurse grabbed his arms and pulled him toward the bed. Harold began thrashing around. Leather restraints were yelled for. He was literally lifted up and thrown onto the bed.

One arm, then the other arm, then both legs were tied securely to the bed frame.

Within minutes Mr. Switek was in full leather restraints, thrashing around the bed, screaming and crying. It was impossible to keep a sheet on the bed or an intravenous line in his arm. Sedation was out of the question because of his lung condition. And the last thing I wanted to do was intubate him again.

He looked at me and yelled, "You can't do this to me! You promised me a cigarette." (He remembered!)

"Mr. Switek, we have to do this," I apologized. "You're going to hurt yourself if we don't keep you here."

He began to sob, the sob of a child, a whimpering for candy denied. I left the room and put in a call for Dr. Janis. I needed help with this man-child, this schizophrenic, tobacco-addicted, emphysema-riddled bull of a patient. I had to keep him from killing himself.

Dr. Janis recommended trying Haldol, a drug less sedating than Thorazine that can be given by intramuscular injection. I agreed. Controlling his psychosis now took priority over his breathing, which was much improved anyway.

Mr. Switek stayed in leather restraints another 36 hours, until the Haldol took effect. Fortunately his breathing remained stable and he was able to take his other medications orally. On the sixth hospital day the leather restraints came off. Miraculously, he had calmed down and was no longer a threat to himself or others.

"Call my mother," he requested.

His mother, old and infirm, had not been able to visit him in MICU. I wanted to speak with her also, so I brought a phone into his room and dialed the number. I handed over the receiver as soon as it began ringing.

"Ma? This is Harold. I'm in the hospital. They're trying to kill me, ma. Yea. They had me all tied up...Yea, they tried to kill me...Bring my cigarettes, OK Ma? I'm coming home now...I don't know, here's the doctor."

I took the receiver from Harold and talked to his mother, a very pleasant lady who, I imagined, had been through some hellish times with her son. She was quite reasonable on the phone. I explained the situation and why her son had to stay in the hospital a little longer and why he could not smoke. She understood and thanked me, adding that she was ready for Harold "whenever you and Dr. Janis say he's ready to come home." We said good bye and I hung up the phone.

"OK, Harold. Your mother says she can't come to see you now but knows you're coming home soon."

He started to cry again. I tried to console him, to reason with him, but it was no use. Mr. Switek was ill in ways I didn't understand and made me feel powerless to help. Since he was not in imminent physical danger I thought it best to just leave him alone.

* * *

The next few days went more smoothly than I expected they would. We gradually weaned down the Haldol dose and switched him back to Thorazine. An arterial blood gas test showed adequate oxygen and carbon dioxide levels. We allowed him to walk outside his room as long as he stayed within the confines of MICU.

By this time a mentally normal patient would have been transferred to a regular ward, but Mr. Switek's psychosis required that he either remain in MICU or go to a psychiatric ward. On the eighth day of hospitalization he returned to Weathergill. During the entire 170 hours in MICU he did not have a single cigarette.

Followup

The above episode took place in 1988. As of this writing Mr. Switek remains on Thorazine and continues to smoke heavily. He has not needed further hospitalization for his lung problem.

12. Pickwickian

I knew Mayzee Fallows for about two years before she was admitted to MICU. I first saw her as an outpatient in 1986 when she was 63. Even then she was enormous — 275 pounds, 5 feet three inches — and had trouble breathing. Her chief complaint was "shortness of my breath."

"Oh Dr. Martin!" she exclaimed back then. "I can't walk from here to there without struggling." She pointed to a wall of my office about 10 feet away.

"How long Mrs. Fallows? How long's it been this bad?"

"Only the past few months. But it seems to get worse each day."

Weight was her problem. Imagine carrying a hundred-pound sack of potatoes packed around your abdomen and rib cage. Just like movement itself, your breathing would be *restricted*. Mayzee breathed this way all the time. Each of her breaths was limited, too shallow to do a proper job of gas exchange.

We normally take in about half a quart of air with each breath. Mayzee could only manage one-forth of a quart. She needed more air but her chest cage couldn't oblige; as a direct result, carbon dioxide in her blood was too high and the oxygen level too low. Mayzee was comfortable at rest but wiped out when walking or climbing stairs.

Breathing difficulty also interrupted her sleep. To compensate, she frequently napped during the day, and at the worst times. She'd had two accidents after falling asleep at the wheel. No one was hurt, including Mayzee, but at age 62 she had to quit driving.

After that first visit I diagnosed Mayzee's problem as typical of Pickwickian syndrome, a triad of obesity, excessive daytime sleepiness, and elevated blood carbon dioxide. To physicians the term 'Pickwickian' connotes a fat, sleepy patient. The name of this curious syndrome comes not from any doctor or patient named Pickwick, but is instead traced to a character in Charles Dickens' first novel, *Pickwick Papers*, published in 1837. At the end of Chapter 53 Dickens introduces a scene involving a fat boy:

A most violent and startling knocking was heard at the door; it was not an ordinary double knock, but a constant and uninterrupted succession of the loudest single raps, as if the knocker were endowed with the perpetual motion, or the person outside had forgotten to leave off...

The object that presented itself to the eyes of the astonished clerk, was a boy - a wonderfully fat boy - habited as a serving lad, standing upright on the mat, with his eyes closed as if in sleep. He had never seen such a fat boy, in or out of a travelling caravan; and this, coupled with the calmness and repose of his appearance, so very different from what was reasonably to have been expected in the inflicter of such knock, smote him with wonder.

"What's the matter" inquired the clerk.

The extraordinary boy replied not a word; but he nodded once, and seemed, to the clerk's imagination, to snore feebly.

"Where do you come from?" inquired the clerk.

The boy made no sign. He breathed heavily, but in all other respects was motionless.

The clerk repeated the question thrice, and receiving no answer, prepared to shut the door, when the boy suddenly opened his eyes, winked several times, sneezed once, and raised his hand as if to repeat the knocking. Finding the door open, he stared about him with astonishment, and at length fixed his eyes on Mr. Lowten's face.

"What the devil do you knock in that way for?" inquired the clerk, angrily.

"Which way?" said the boy, in a slow and sleepy voice.

"Why, like forty hackney-coachmen," replied the clerk.

"Because master said, I wasn't to leave off knocking till they opened the door, for fear I should go to sleep," said the boy.

Dickens's portrayal lay dormant medically for 119 years, until 1956 when Dr. C.S. Burwell and colleagues published a medical case report titled "Extreme obesity associated with alveolar hypoventilation — a Pickwickian syndrome." After quoting Dickens's description of the fat boy, the authors went on to describe their patient, a 51-year-old business executive who stood 5 feet 5 inches and weighed over 260 pounds:

[He] entered the hospital because of obesity, fatigue and somnolence... The patient was accustomed to eating well but did not gain weight progressively until about one year before admission... As the patient gained weight his symptoms appeared and became worse..he had often fallen asleep while carrying on his daily routine...on several occasions he suffered brief episodes of syncope [fainting]. Persistent edema of the ankles developed... Finally an experience which indicated the severity of his disability led him to seek hospital care. The patient was accustomed to playing poker once a week and on this crucial occasion he was dealt a hand of three aces and two kings. According to Hoyle this hand is called a "full house." *Because he had dropped off to sleep he failed to take advantage of this opportunity.* [Italics original]. A few days later he entered...hospital.

"...Therapy consisted chiefly of enforced weight reduction by means of an 800-calory diet. On this regimen the patient's weight fell from 121.4 to 103.6 kg [267 to 228 pounds] in a period of three weeks. As he lost weight his somnolence, twitching, periodic respiration, dyspnea and edema gradually subsided and his physical condition became essentially normal."

Since that first medical paper thousands of patients have been diagnosed with sleep disorders. The spectrum of problems ranges from occasional insomnia to sleep walking to the far more serious and potentially life-threatening Pickwickian syndrome. Many hospitals run "sleep labs," secluded rooms replete with bed and exotic monitoring equipment for charting physiology during sleep.

Mayzee Fallows needed such an evaluation. More important, she needed to lose weight. Even if her sleep pattern tested normal, which I knew it wouldn't, her weight was a serious problem.

Mayzee's wedding picture at 23 showed a woman of 140 lbs, solid and attractive. By age 50 she tipped the scales at 200 lbs but had no (known) medical problems. At 60 she weighed 240 lbs and was under treatment for high blood pressure and diabetes. She added another 35 pounds over the next three years. Fortunately Mayzee did not smoke (the combination of cigarettes and morbid obesity would have been fatal well before I ever saw her). As it was, she could barely manage.

Why did she eat all that food?

"I don't eat that much." she said. "Honest I don't, Dr. Martin."

Doctors used to discount this claim, heard from many massively obese people, but to a certain extent it may be true. Metabolism nose dives in middle age and a normal or even slightly-low calorie diet may not bring about any weight loss, at least not without added exercise. But daily, aerobic-type exercise for people like Mayzee Fallows is simply not feasible. The only solution for the massively obese is such a drastic decrease in calories that medical supervision becomes necessary.

Mayzee had been on diets before but they always failed. No will power, she confessed. She had never been in a medically-supervised weight loss program.

"Mayzee," I said, "you need two things. First, you need to lose weight in a special program so doctors can follow your metabolism. And we need to study your breathing to see why your oxygen is so low. The only way to do both is put you in the hospital."

"Hospital? It's that bad?"

"Yes," I insisted.

"Will my insurance cover it?"

I checked. Her insurance plan did not recognize hospitalization for obesity alone, so I admitted her for "respiratory failure, chronic." Unfortunately for Mayzee this was a legitimate diagnosis, confirmed by the elevated carbon dioxide level in her blood.

We did a battery of tests to check function of her heart, lungs, liver, kidneys, pancreas, and adrenal glands. Surprisingly, everything checked out normal or near-normal except her lungs. Lung function tests showed severe 'restrictive' impairment, confirming the clinical impression. As a result of shallow breathing the oxygen pressure in her blood was reduced to 55 (normal is above 85) and carbon dioxide pressure was elevated to 53 (normal is between 36 and 44). Some physicians would say that Mayzee belonged to the '50-50' club, referring to her O_2 and

CO_2 levels. Membership is definitely not desirable.

On the evening of day three routine tests were completed and she was sent to a another wing of the hospital for a sleep study, technically known as 'polysomnography' (literally, the recording of many (poly) records (graphy) during sleep (somno)). The studies are conducted in a windowless room with the patient laying on a queen-sized bed (large enough to accommodate the heaviest patients). After Mayzee lay down technicians connected wires, emanating from various monitoring devices, to her head, nose, ear, chest, and extremities.

I went to observe the beginning of her sleep study. Laying flat, wired up, and surrounded by all kinds of electronic boxes, Mayzee looked like a character in a sci-fi thriller. I thought of taking a picture and sending it to one of the national tabloids. The headline would blare **FAT WOMAN ZAPPED INTO THIN BEAUTY**, or something like that. My picture would be the 'before' pose. The tabloid would find a beautiful model with a similar face for the after shot. (I didn't do it, of course, but just remember where the idea originated.)

Twenty minutes later Mayzee was fast asleep and I left her to the sleep technician. Mayzee slept from 10 p.m. to 6:30 a.m., at which time she was taken back to her regular ward bed. I saw her on morning rounds.

"Well, Mrs. Fallows, did you sleep last night?"

"Sure did, Dr. Martin. All those wires didn't bother me a bit."

"Don't you feel tired?"

"No, not right now."

I went to the sleep lab to check the results. The tests showed three things. Mayzee snored a lot; her throat tended to close and block her upper airway during sleep; and her blood oxygen fell, at one point to 38, a level not compatible with long life. She was at risk for *sudden death.*

I prescribed a plastic gizmo that fits over the nose and forces a continuous stream of air into the throat. Called 'nasal CPAP,' the device is only worn by the patient during sleep. The continuous jet of air keeps the upper airway from closing and, in many patients, the oxygen level from falling. Mayzee tried the nasal CPAP only two nights before rejecting it. "It's like sleeping in an air vent," she said.

I gave her a more acceptable nasal cannula for use during sleep; it delivers extra oxygen through the nostrils, but at no increase in air pressure. The oxygen at least kept her O_2 level from hitting rock bottom while she slept.

In the middle of week two Mayzee started the Optifast protein supplement diet. In this diet all food is taken away and the patient drinks only a liquid protein supplement several times a day. The supplement allows the body to burn mainly carbohydrate and fat during what amounts to semi-starvation. For patients who stick to the supplement there is often remarkable — and safe — weight loss.

After three weeks in hospital Mayzee went home weighing 255 pounds. A 20 pound weight loss was not bad in such a short period, but the first 20 are the easiest. Now all she had to do was continue the diet, plus use oxygen at night.

At first all was success. A month after discharge she weighed 240 pounds and her oxygen level was up. Two months after discharge she weighed 230 pounds, a satisfying drop of 45 pounds in only three months. She looked and felt better and had improved blood gases as well.

But alas, something happened. She quit attending the clinic. Since that was the only place to get the protein supplement, she quit dieting as well. About a month afterwards I received a card from Optifast Clinic: 'Your patient, MAYZEE FALLOWS, has dropped out of the Optifast Program. Please let us know if we can be of any further help in her weight control.'

I called the patient. "Mrs. Fallows, what happened? Why did you quit going to Optifast?"

"Oh, Dr. Martin. I couldn't get a ride anymore. And it was just too far by bus."

People who lose weight in the best of programs frequently gain it back. Reasons for sliding are varied, but Mayzee's was a common one — inability to keep up clinic appointments. She could have found other transportation but didn't make the effort.

On the phone she admitted to gaining weight and having more trouble breathing. I saw her the next day, in my office at the hospital. She weighed 262 pounds and had leg edema (swelling from excess fluid). A chest x-ray confirmed early congestive heart failure. I admitted her to the hospital and began diuretics to mobilize the fluid. She did not need the intensive care unit on this admission.

Our specialist in morbid obesity saw her in consultation. He didn't mince words. "Given the severity of her problem and recent failure on the Optifast diet, I suggest consideration for gastric stapling. Please contact Surgery."

First you try dieting without supervision. That seldom works. Then you try supervised dieting. That is sometimes successful. When it fails you have a range of procedures to choose from, all disappointing in their long term results. Gastric stapling, literally stapling the stomach into a smaller pouch for receiving food, is one of the more popular operations for the massively obese. The 'stapled' stomach is supposed to make the patient feel satiated with less food. Success with the operation is limited, however. Perhaps a quarter of the patients maintain significant weight reduction over the long term.

A surgeon visited Mayzee to explain the operation and the risks. "Let me think about it," she said. She thought about the procedure for two days and decided against it. "I'll lose weight with the diet," she said.

"Mayzee," I remarked on learning of her decision, "you failed the diet. You gave up."

"Oh, Dr. Martin! I won't quit next time. I promise."

"It's up to you, Mayzee."

"Let me try again," she said.

She was accepted back into the Optifast program. We also made special arrangements for transportation if she couldn't find a ride to the clinic. Most patients are given only two chances in the program; this was Mayzee's second.

She left the hospital in a week, weighing 253 pounds.

*   *   *

Mayzee quit the Optifast diet three months later, this time with the excuse that "it just wasn't for me." Compliance is everything in weight reduction and there was nothing more the

Optifast Clinic could do.

She continued using the oxygen cannula and diuretics, and her weight did not go down. It didn't go up either, but age was against her. What the 30- or 40- or 50-year-old-body can tolerate, the 64- or 65-year-old can find unbearable.

I followed Mayzee, along with her internist, but we could not correct her underlying medical problems. Her oxygen and carbon dioxide levels remained grossly out of balance. She was — I told her several times — a ticking time bomb. It was a question of when, not if.

The bomb went off late in March, 1988, just after she turned 65. I was called from the emergency room. "Dr. Martin, this is Dr. T. I understand you know Mayzee Fallows? Her internist asked that I contact you."

"Yes, yes. What happened?"

"Mrs. Fallows rolled in about an hour ago, almost apneic. We intubated her and will be sending her up to MICU."

"I was afraid this would happen. What caused her decompensation?"

"We don't know. Chest x-ray's clear and her cardiogram shows no acute changes. She apparently collapsed at home and EMS [Emergency Medical Service] was called. When she got here her PCO-two was ninety-six, and PO-two thirty-five."

"Wow! Sounds like she was on her way out."

"Yes. We had real trouble intubating her. Finally had to go through her nose. Her blood gases are improving on the ventilator and she's stable enough to be moved. Do you have a bed available?"

"Sure. Send her right up."

I *thought* I knew Mayzee but the person rolled into MICU was much larger than what I remembered. She must have gained another 50 pounds. Three nurses and two doctors lifted her from the transport stretcher to hospital bed. HEAVY.

Her MICU bed rested on a scale so that additional weight could be accurately recorded. She weighed 318 lbs. and looked it. Her belly was enormous. How could anyone breathe with all that fat pressing on her lungs?

About an hour later, after things were squared away with Mrs.

Fallows, I went to talk to Mr. Fallows in the family waiting area. Thin, in his mid-60's, he had just recently retired from a job with the post office. I knew from previous visits that their marriage was a good one and that Mr. Fallows was devoted to her care. Unfortunately there was little he could do without her cooperation.

"She's stable now, Mr. Fallows," I said. "But she was in a lot of trouble when she arrived here. What happened to her? Look's like she's gained over 50 pounds since I last saw her."

"I don't know, Doctor Martin. She just lays around at home and doesn't do much. For the last few days she's been kind of mopy. Today I couldn't even get her out of bed."

"Why didn't you call us before?"

"She didn't want to come to the hospital. She told me not to call the ambulance. Said she was fine, just wanted to be left alone."

I affirmed that she was critically ill and could die any time.

"Well, I have faith. Just do what you can for her, Dr. Martin."

Our initial tests did not reveal any acute infection or other explanation for Mrs. Fallows' deterioration. She seemed to have worsened just from increase in both age and weight. That left only weight to correct. Until we took off a couple dozen pounds — or redistributed them — she would likely need the ventilator.

The next morning on rounds we found her awake, laying in bed with her head raised slightly on one pillow. She looked pachydermish with the endotracheal tube coming our of her right nostril, a giant, thick neck, and a mountain of fat south of that. Her legs were huge, rounded limbs of hardened tissue, the result of years of edema. The skin around her ankles was bluish-red and scaly.

I arranged the sheets to reveal her abdominal protuberance. We've had heavier patients before (one of 550 lbs), but Mayzee's short stature and roly poly appearance made her somehow look more grotesque than our others. Clinical observation and professionalism aside, such patients always elicit a bit of voyeurism. So it was on rounds. Everyone stared at Mayzee's belly.

Putting my hands on her huge abdomen, I said: *"This* is the problem." Mrs. Fallows nodded in agreement. "I'm not going to minimize the situation, Mayzee. Your weight is killing you. It's got to come off." She nodded again.

"We'll do what we can to get that tube out of your nose. But when we do, you have to lose some weight. Or you'll be right back here." I pointed to her bed and she nodded.

I went over the ventilator settings and blood gases with the house staff, examined Mayzee's lungs and heart, reviewed her fluid intake and urine output. She was stable but not ready to come off the ventilator. I led the housestaff out of her room, to resume our discussion in the hallway.

"What would you do now?" I asked Sherry, one of the interns.

"I don't know. Can we keep her on the ventilator while she loses weight? I guess that's one way to stop her from eating."

"Is there any alternative? Can we get her off the ventilator the way she is now?"

The group was stumped.

"What's her major problem?" I asked.

"Her weight."

"Right. Any other problem?"

"Well, hypertension."

"Right, that's a problem too, but it's not what I'm thinking. Is there any other reason she could be in respiratory failure besides the weight?"

"She doesn't smoke and has no asthma. Her chest X-ray is clear. What are you getting at, Dr. Martin?"

"Suppose you studied blood gases and breathing capacity in 20 non-smokers under 5 feet 3 inches and weighing over 300 pounds. What do you think you would find?"

"I don't know," said Sherry. "Did you do that study?"

"No, but others have. There are minor abnormalities in some people, but in most the breathing capacity and blood gases are normal or at least near normal, even in people over age 60. The point is, weight by itself is not the only problem. There has to be another factor or factors to explain *her* problem. I've been following Mrs. Fallows for two years. Even when her weight was two-fifty she had trouble with oxygen and carbon dioxide.

"Most likely patients like Mrs. Fallows have an abnormal

brainstem respiratory center. For some reason, her brain won't let her do the extra work of breathing all that extra weight requires. Many obese people *are* able to do the extra work and maintain good oxygen and CO-two levels. She doesn't do the extra work necessary for deeper breaths, so her blood gases are abnormal. It's just a theory, but it does help explain why not every obese person has Mrs. Fallows's problem."

"Would respiratory stimulants help?" asked Sherry.

"You mean some kind of pill to stimulate her brain stem?"

"Yes, something like that."

"A few have been tried, particularly progesterone. They generally don't work, and if they do it's only over the long term. Certainly that's not going to help in the short term. We've got to get her off the ventilator very soon. Any ideas?"

"Besides cutting it off?" Laughter.

"Why can't we do a fat-ectomy?"

"What about wiring her jaw shut?"

"You laugh," I said, "but all those are possibilities. Still, you're not answering my question. How can we safely remove her from the ventilator in the next few days? She's not going to lose enough weight to make a big difference in a few days. How are we going to do it?"

"Diuretics."

"They will help mobilize excess water, but probably won't make much of a dent in her belly. She's already on Lasix [a potent diuretic]. Any other ideas?"

No answer.

"Well, there's one way," I said. "A therapy too little used in MICU. What?"

They were stumped by my guess-what-I'm-thinking question.

"I'll give you a hint. It's not a drug and not a medical device."

"What else is there?" asked Sherry.

"I'll give you another hint. It's an elemental force of nature. One of the four primary forces."

"Ohhhhhhh," said the medical resident, who had been listening intently.

"Yes?"

"Newton."

"That's right. We're going to use *gravity*. It's free and every room is equipped. If we don't get that tube out of her throat soon she's bound to have a major complication. Infection or airway damage. A tracheostomy on Mrs. Fallows will be very difficult. She has no neck. A surgeon looking for a hole in her trachea could get lost." The housestaff stared at Mayzee through the glass doors; there was no arguing my point. "We've got to get her off the ventilator," I said. "The only way is with...an anti-gravity bed."

"What's that?"

"A bed that will allow her to sit up without sliding to the floor. Look at her. She's in the anti-breathing position. Her abdomen is like a sack of potatoes pushing on her chest. How can she breathe on her own? If we can just unload her lungs I think we can her off the ventilator."

"Marsha," I said to our head nurse, "can we get her one of those Big Boy beds? You know, the kind we used before on that five-hundred pounder?"

"Sure, Dr. Martin. I'll see what I can do."

*   *   *

Unlike a conventional hospital bed, the Big Boy is constructed in sections. Each section can be raised or lowered to bend the patient in whatever position desired. With the Big Boy we were able to raise Mrs. Fallows' chest at an angle of 60 degrees from her abdomen. At the same time we kept her legs stretched out to a comfortable, near-horizontal position. This posture effectively shifted her massive abdomen away from the chest and gave her lungs more room to expand with each breath. She remained this way (with slight variation) for the next two days while we gradually turned down the ventilator settings.

On her third MICU day we disconnected Mayzee from the ventilator, leaving the endotracheal tube in place. At that point she breathed on her own, through the tube. Her arterial blood gases remained about the same as baseline values: PO_2 64, PCO_2 59. I decided to take a chance and pull the endotracheal tube. We could always put it back in.

After extubation Mayzee's PO$_2$ remained borderline low, PCO$_2$ high. Although she did not need re-intubation she wasn't ready to leave MICU either. I would describe her state as a 'ventilatory limbo,' almost-but-not quite needing artificial ventilation, almost-but-not quite ready to leave MICU for a regular ward bed.

When not sleeping Mayzee just laid in bed. She made few demands on the nurses and generally seemed unconcerned about her situation. There was no hint of desire to get better and leave MICU. Had she given up? Or was her mood a result of deranged blood gases? We found no evidence for neurologic damage. She was oriented and conversant but just seemed unmotivated. Overall, a bad sign.

Mayzee's fifth day in hospital, April 1, was also the day house staff changed rotations. Her new intern was Roger Bailes, a 29-year-old with a career interest in emergency medicine. Dr. Bailes was in his ninth month of internship (the academic year begins in July) and he had already spent a month in MICU in October. He knew his way around. What he didn't know, unfortunately, was much pulmonary physiology.

Interns and residents cannot choose their patients. They have to take whoever is assigned to them and Mayzee came under Dr. Bailes' care. Unfortunately he wasn't very sympathetic to her condition. As far as he was concerned, if she just took deeper breaths she could get out of MICU and off his service. He didn't like obese, slothful patients.

During morning rounds on April 3 he asked, "Dr. Martin, can we transfer her out of MICU today? I don't think we're doing much for her here."

"What's her blood gas this morning?" I asked.

"About the same. PCO-two is seventy-two, PO-two fifty-six, on nasal oxygen."

I reviewed all the blood gases obtained since extubation. They did not show much variation: chronic hypoventilation [underbreathing] and low oxygen levels. We had tried everything to improve her gas exchange, including sitting her up in the Big Boy bed, deep breathing exercises, adjustments of diet, and diuretics to mobilize edema fluid.

"I don't know," I said wistfully. "I wish she could just take deeper breaths and lower her CO-two."

At my remark Dr. Bailes' eyes opened wide. He must have been looking for the proper opening and I provided it. "I think I have an explanation for her failure to improve," he said.

"Really? What?"

"Mrs. Fallows just doesn't want to breathe more. It's her personality. She needs more motivation." Translation: psychiatry consult and transfer out of MICU. Not a bad idea on the surface, but incredibly naive *in her case*. I decided to respond with mock incredulity.

"WHAT? What did you say? It's her personality?"

"Yes," he replied seriously. "Some patients just don't want to breathe deeply. She's just lazy and wants to be this way. Maybe psychiatry can help her."

How to answer this medical delusion? He was so wrong I was actually amused. Personality and attitude have nothing — NOTHING — to do with why patients underbreathe or have a low oxygen level. Nobel-prize winning physiology showed long ago that you cannot will yourself to hypoventilate or become hypoxemic (transcendental meditation notwithstanding). That is why children who hold their breath to gain attention cannot harm themselves. The brain won't let a child — or an adult — voluntarily slow down breathing to a dangerous level.

I decided to give Dr. Bailes benefit of doubt. Perhaps I misunderstood his meaning. "You mean because she eats a lot that her breathing is affected, and that Psychiatry could help motivate her to lose weight. Is that what you mean?" I asked.

"Well, that too." said Roger. "But you see this kind of breathing in lazy people. It's just her basic personality."

'Wow!' I thought. Was he putting me on?

"Roger, do you have a reference for that?"

"Well, I read that somewhere," he said lamely.

"Where?"

"I don't remember. Somewhere."

I went on the attack.

"Roger, what's the average PCO-two of patients on the psychiatry ward?"

"I don't know," he said.

"Anybody?"

"Forty?" asked Sherry.

"Forty point oh oh," I said. "Normal."

"Now, what's the average PCO-two of prison inmates?" No one answered.

"Forty point oh oh. Normal. And what is the average PCO-two of all the people who are nasty, mean, uncivilized, and LAZY?"

This time I refused to answer my own question.

"Forty?" said Sherry again.

"Right. Forty point oh oh. Any other bad traits you want to know about as far as the associated PCO-two?" It was all in good fun. No one seemed offended and the other housestaff, at least, were enjoying the exercise.

"Roger," I continued, "you clearly don't know what can make someone hypoventilate. Fat can do it. She's fat. Lesions in the brainstem can do it. That's a theorectical possibility and no good way to prove it. Long term smoking can do it but she doesn't smoke. Some drugs can slow your breathing but she's not on any of those. Muscle weakness can do it and she may have that. But personality? Never."

No one said anything. Time for the old repetition routine. If you can't help the patient, at least teach the housestaff. Make a point so they'll *never forget*, even if you have to make yourself seem obnoxious in the process. "Sherry, can a patient's personality explain an elevated CO-two level?"

At first Sherry looked startled, then she caught on. "No, Dr. Martin. Personality can't be blamed."

"Roger, can the nature of a patient's personality explain an elevated CO-two?"

He took my obnoxious question good-naturedly. "No, Dr. Martin, personality can't be blamed."

"OK. Anybody have any questions?" No one did.

"Well," I said, "I think we've done everything possible for Mrs. Fallows in MICU. Why don't we transfer her upstairs."

Followup

Mrs. Fallows stayed in the hospital another two weeks. Her attitude improved along with a return to ambulation. On the day of discharge her weight was down 45 pounds and arterial blood gases were better than in MICU, though still not normal.

She was given a rare third chance in the Optifast Program. She stayed with the diet for a few months, then stopped a third time. Two months later she collapsed at home. Mr. Fallows called Emergency Medical Service and paramedics reached the house within minutes. They found her apneic and began CPR, which was continued during the ten minute ambulance ride to the hospital. On arrival in the emergency room she had no pulse except that provided by chest compressions. Another half hour of CPR failed to restore her heart beat and she was pronounced dead. No autopsy was performed.

13. Coma

There is coma and there is COMA. Jack Wilkerson, a 35-year-old accountant, was out for six months and we never knew why. His case was the stuff of tabloids (**MAN SLEEPS HALF-YEAR — DOCS BAFFLED**) and also the kind that ends up in medical journals ('Prolonged coma of unknown etiology: report of a case and review of the literature').

It happened this way. One day in July I got a call from the emergency room. "Dr. Martin, we have a 35 year-old man who may have encephalitis. He's confused and febrile to one hundred point two. His brother says it began with a headache last night and this morning he didn't know where he was."

"Has be been tapped?" I asked.

"Yes, his spinal tap is clear, so we don't think he has meningitis. Anyway, he's going for a CAT scan and then to MICU."

Apart from the fact that encephalitis is always a serious medical problem, there was nothing particularly unique or startling about this message. We see encephalitis all the time. Because of the potential for disaster, such as respiratory failure, everyone with this diagnosis is first admitted to the medical intensive care unit.

On arrival to MICU Jack Wilkerson did not look ill at all, just a bit drowsy and confused. Of average height and stocky, he had a day's growth of beard and a sweet, round face that tended to stare off into space, both eyes wide open. He was arousable by shaking, and actually answered some questions appropriately, but for others his answers made no sense.

"What's your name?"

"Jack."

"Jack what?"

"Jack."

"Where are you, Jack?"

"My brother."

"Anything hurt you, Jack?"

"Yes."

"What?"

"Yes."

And so it went. All we knew was that Mr. Wilkerson had been healthy two days earlier, and that along with his confusional state he had a fever but no evidence for meningitis (inflammation of membranes surrounding the brain). Instead, the clinical picture suggested encephalitis or inflammation *within* the brain. His vital signs were stable and otherwise he seemed in good physical health.

Additional medical history provided by his brother was not especially helpful. The patient had never been sick before: tonsils out at age eleven, occasional flu syndrome, but no illnesses of any type for about a year. He was a certified public accountant and lived alone. He was unmarried but had no history of homosexuality. Nor was there any history of drug abuse or alcoholism or travel outside the country. In short, nothing to suggest a diagnosis more specific than "encephalitis of unknown cause."

The CAT scan of his brain was negative: no evidence for stroke, hemorrhage, or tumor. We ordered blood cultures and many other blood tests; all eventually came back normal or negative. A 'toxic screen' of his blood — a test for about a dozen common poisons and drugs people overdose on — turned up nothing except aspirin, and at a level expected in someone using the drug for headache. Urine and feces were examined for infecting organisms; none were found. Blood was sent to the state lab for viral titers; these results would be inconclusive until repeat testing could be accomplished in three weeks to check for a diagnostic rise in titer.

Six hours after admission to MICU Jack became less responsive. His level of breathing remained adequate but his eyes were now closed, a sign of developing coma. A plastic catheter was inserted into his radial artery so arterial blood could be drawn to monitor oxygen and carbon dioxide. Another tube was inserted through his penis into his bladder, to monitor urine output.

Mr. Wilkerson deteriorated rapidly. Twelve hours after he first presented his breathing became shallow and his blood carbon dioxide level began to rise. Respiratory failure set in. To provide artificial ventilation doctors inserted a foot-long hollow plastic endotracheal tube into his windpipe, and connected it to the ventilator. Until coma reversed the patient would have to be breathed by machine.

Another tube was inserted through his nose and into the stomach, for feeding. Twenty-four hours after hospital admission Jack Wilkerson had five plastic tubes in his body and was completely comatose.

We called in two consultants, Neurology and Infectious Disease. "Stage IV coma — possible encephalitis," opined the former. "Recommend continued support. Check titers for possible viral etiology."

The ID specialist was no more helpful. "Puzzling case, not typical of encephalitis in this area. No indication for antibiotic coverage." (Note to medical readers; this case pre-dated current antibiotic therapy for some types of viral encephalitis).

Mr. Wilkerson's coma continued. More doctors came by, to ponder or wonder or offer their advice. It all amounted to the same thing: wait and watch.

The second week came and went, without improvement. The toll was especially hard on Jack's brother. Tom Wilkerson, 38, owned a cabinet shop, had a wife and two kids, and was as close to his brother as any adult sibling could be. Tom's business suffered as he spent hours at Jack's bedside. "When do you think my brother will wake up? Anything new?" Always the same good questions and always the same answer — 'We don't know.'

The longer someone is in coma the worse the prognosis. This is not necessarily because the brain is damaged, but because the rest of the body tends to wither from disuse, particularly the arm and leg muscles. Also, bed sores develop quickly unless the patient is regularly turned from side to side.

The many plastic tubes necessary for medical care can also cause problems. The urinary tract becomes ripe for infection with a catheter in the bladder. The endotracheal tube can damage the vocal cords and trachea. Catheters in the arteries and veins tend to cause inflammation and infection if not meticulously cared for and changed frequently. Also, because of inadequate nutrition body weight almost always falls in the comatose patient; a feeding tube is no substitute for the healthy appetite.

A completely comatose patient requires a small army of nurses and therapists to prevent complications of lying still for so long. Around the clock people had to turn Mr. Wilkerson from side to side, massage his muscles, change his catheters, oil his skin, feed his stomach. It would do no good to have him wake up only to be crippled by muscle contractions, or missing a limb from hospital-acquired infection, or suffering a giant decubitus ulcer (these things have happened).

Jack's body was well maintained. As for his brain, it had its own agenda. He did not wake up. There was not even a glimmer of improvement. A brain wave test — electroencephalogram — was carried out once a week but it's pattern never varied: "...slow waves consistent with encephalopathy." No diagnosis, really.

At Tom's suggestion, and with our ready acquiescence, a consultant neurologist was called in from another hospital, someone no more qualified than our own staff neurologist but perhaps able to offer a fresh perspective. His conclusion after two hours with the patient and the chart: "Agree with current management. Continue what you are doing."

Mr. Wilkerson's case became part of the hospital's culture. I was no longer met in the hallway with the perfunctory 'How are you doing?' but with 'How's Mr. Wilkerson doing?' "The same," I found myself replying each time. "Still sleeping."

By the middle of the third week, when it became clear Mr. Wilkerson was not going to wake up soon, he went for tracheostomy. This operation places a short breathing tube directly through the neck into the trachea, and is routine for patients who require prolonged artificial ventilation. It frees up the mouth and provides for much better oral hygiene. Also, if the patient is awake he or she can eat while being breathed by machine.

During the fourth week we took out Jack's nasogastric feeding tube. To provide a better conduit for food surgeons placed a rubber feeding tube directly through his abdominal skin into the stomach, a procedure called percutaneous endoscopic gastrostomy (PEG). With both the endotracheal and feeding tubes removed

Mr. Wilkerson looked much more comfortable. Whether he felt that way was impossible to know.

By the end of a month all his tubes had been changed at least once, some as many as five times. His weight was down from 180 pounds on admission to 147, and holding steady. Every-other-day blood tests showed no deterioration of any vital organ. In short, Mr. Wilkerson was stable, just not recovering from coma.

Repeat viral titers were sent to the state lab. To our surprise, all tested negative; there was no rise in titer of any virus known to cause encephalitis in our state.

Mr. Wilkerson's case was explored in conference after conference at the hospital. The ID people presented his problem in a seminar on difficult-to-diagnose encephalitis. The neurologists found his length and and depth of coma worthy of academic discourse. Lung specialists waxed over the subject of prolonged artificial ventilation. Nurses discussed basic care of the unconscious patient, and the physical therapists highlighted the importance of maintaining muscle tone by passive range of motion. The nutritionists talked about feeding the comatose patient and assured us (as we already knew) that, food-wise, Jack could be kept alive "forever."

A month elapsed and still there was no improvement. Emboldened by his survival yet dismayed by the lack of progress, we decided it was time to experiment. Perhaps something in our patient's blood was causing coma that we could not detect with all our tests. A method is available for 'washing' the blood of unwanted proteins, called 'plasmapheresis.' Had plasmapheresis ever been used before in prolonged coma? Well, no, at least not at our hospital. But it is used successfully in other afflictions of the nervous system, including Guillain Barré syndrome and myasthenia gravis. True, these are disorders of the *peripheral nervous system*, not the brain, but what did we have to lose? What did Jack Wilkerson have to lose? Because the procedure was somewhat experimental, at least in this case, we asked for and readily received permission from his brother.

Three times a week the plasmapheresis device, a bulky machine the size of a console TV, was wheeled into his room and connected via tubing to his arm veins. Blood from one vein entered the machine to be "pheresed," or washed, and a fresh plasma-like solution was instilled back into another vein. Each washing session lasted about two hours. From experience with other diseases a beneficial effect from pheresis might not be seen for weeks.

We continued plasmapheresis for a whole month, longer than usual in other diseases. Mr. Wilkerson didn't get worse and he didn't get better. Essentially nothing happened.

At the end of the plasmapheresis trial — after two months in the hospital — I noticed a perceptible shift in attitude among the hospital staff. Many now felt that Mr. Wilkerson would never wake up, that he wasn't going to live. This attitude found its way into the hospital chart, among notes of the several consultants still involved in his care: "Prognosis appears hopeless" and "At this point doubt meaningful recovery" and "Poor outlook. Discussed with brother."

No one actually gave up, of course. He continued to receive excellent care. But the clinical and intellectual excitement of the first two months was no longer present, and other patients and other problems took center stage. Jack Wilkerson's coma became more or less an accepted fact and his problem was pushed 'to the back' of the ICU. We continued daily bedside rounds but his blood was now drawn only once a week, a chest x-ray taken only every ten days or so, and the chart notes became less wordy and appeared less often.

"About the same."

"No change today."

"Vital signs stable."

Only the intern, newly assigned each month, wrote comprehensive notes. Everyone else sort of backed off. This change in intensity of care was entirely appropriate. We had done virtually everything feasible and, apart from supporting his ventilation and monitoring bodily functions, as physicians we seemed to have no therapeutic role. If Mr. Wilkerson was going to wake up it would be on his brain's own timetable.

Tom Wilkerson never gave up. He was at his brother's side daily, talking to him, reading letters, playing the radio. It is a matter of controversy whether comatose patients benefit from stimulation by familiar sounds. Tom had discussed the issue with several laymen and was convinced of the value of audio stimulation. We were more than happy to go along with this and made sure that Jack "listened" to music via headphones at least six hours a day.

Fall came and went. Discussions were held about sending Mr. Wilkerson to a chronic care facility but his brother was against it. He felt Jack's only chance was to remain in the hospital, in the ICU.

The new year came. We had no plans to move him or change anything, just to continue administering food, fluids, artificial ventilation, and good nursing care. No one expected anything more.

*   *   *

One day in mid January, as suddenly as it had begun, Jack's coma lifted. He opened his eyes and looked at a nurse washing his face. I was not there but heard that she cried out, "Jack, you're awake!"

Because of the tracheostomy tube he could not talk even if he remembered how, but he was evidently coherent. He looked around, as if to ask "Where am I?" Everyone came to see and stare. One nurse remarked, not inappropriately, that it was like seeing a dead man wake up.

Suddenly the chart notes blossomed. "Mr. Wilkerson appears to have spontaneously recovered from prolonged coma," wrote the neurologist. "Will repeat EEG."

"Spontaneous remission of ?non-infectious encephalitis," wrote the ID specialist.

"Remarkable improvement," wrote the intern in her daily note.

"Praise God," said Jack's brother, not usually taken to religious commentary. "What made him come out of it?"

"I don't know. No one knows!" I exclaimed. "Let's hope he doesn't relapse." That is always a possibility with encephalitis.

It took another week to get Mr. Wilkerson off the breathing machine, then several more days to get him to the point of standing at the bedside. Remarkably, amazingly, he continued to improve, haltingly at first, then steadily, with each passing day.

After two weeks of aggressive physical therapy he learned to walk again. The whole hospital turned out to observe. And to enjoy.

*   *   *

One day in early February Jack was wheeled down to the lobby where his brother's car was waiting to take him home. Using a cane for balance and helped by his brother and a hospital aid, but walking under his own power, Jack entered the front seat of the car and the door closed. He had been hospitalized seven months and three days.

Extensive neurologic testing in April revealed no significant deficits. His EEG was read as normal and residual muscle weakness we attributed to prolonged disuse rather than any nerve damage. He returned to his accounting job and reported no problems with memory or calculating ability. By May Jack Wilkerson was back working a 40-hour week.

Several years after admission for prolonged coma, Jack Wilkerson is healthy and well.

Comment

Jack Wilkerson's recall of seven months in the hospital *begins* with his first trip to physical therapy, about a week after he woke up. The entire hospital stay until that point is a blank. He feels lucky to be alive and, like the rest of us, has no idea what happened or why.

Many people cite his case as an example of why doctors should never give up on a patient in coma, but it is often a comparison of apples to oranges. Mr. Wilkerson's problem was coma of unknown cause in an otherwise healthy body. The outlook is very different for many known causes of coma, such as with the patient in the next story.

14. Cocaine Wins

Lester Brown was a large man, at least 6 feet 2 inches and 240 pounds. Even asleep he looked menacingly big, someone you didn't want to wake up before he was ready. The day he came to MICU you could have shook and pinched and tickled Mr. Brown and he wouldn't bother you. He had a ruptured blood vessel at the base of his brain.

It started at home. A few minutes after inhaling some cocaine his posterior communicating cerebral artery began to pulsate, causing him to complain of "the worst headache of my life." Seconds later he fell to the floor, unconscious. En route to the emergency room the artery burst and he suffered a full blown *subarachnoid hemorrhage*. The loss of an ounce of blood relieved the pressure within his artery and the hemorrhage ceased but by then it was too late. Irritating blood washed over the normally smooth brain surfaces where it didn't belong, and in the process shut down his central nervous system's reticular activating system and put Lester Brown into a deep coma.

Mr. Brown was 41 years old and had been using cocaine for six or seven years. Like all cocaine-related knockouts, Lester's occurred not from a steady accretion of drug but from a single, exciting snort. Within 30 minutes after inhaling the cocaine he was in Memorial Medical Center's emergency room, comatose and intubated, his breathing supported by a ventilator.

A CAT scan of his brain confirmed the clinical diagnosis. It showed blood everywhere, both within the ventricles of the brain and covering the outside surfaces. From CAT scan he was sent to MICU and both neurosurgery and neurology consultants were immediately called.

His brother, three years younger but equally large and sinister looking as Lester, gave us the history. 'Buba' Brown made no attempt to hide his and Lester's illicit activity; indeed, he recounted the details as if we knew all along about their habit and drug trade.

"We just did our thing, man, and this happened. We didn't try to hurt no one. We just dealt with dudes we didn't know too well. Shit, man, this could've happened to me. Mother Fuckers!"

Although Lester's hemorrhage was explainable by a sudden whiff of pure coke — a well-documented occurrence in cocaine users — his brother believed in a more sinister cause. "I told him not to buy off those guys. Lester, he didn't think he had enemies. Man, what are you going to do. I can't believe this happened to Lester. Mother fuckers!"

"What do you think they sold him?" I asked, more out of curiosity about the drug trade than belief that the answer would affect Lester's outcome.

"Never you mind," Buba said. "I know. And they know I know. Is he gonna make it? I mean, that's what I need to know now, Doc, is he gonna make it?"

"It's too early to tell but it doesn't look good. The neurosurgeon and neurologist are on their way to see him."

* * *

It is axiomatic that all patients are treated *without discrimination* in intensive care units. The physical space, the level of nursing care, indeed the entire resources of the hospital are the same for all ICU patients. This *equal level* is not always true elsewhere in the hospital, where there can be distinctions between single vs. private rooms, private duty vs. staff nursing, care by private physicians only vs. care by salaried physicians, etc. In the ICU it doesn't matter if you are a pauper or king, drug addict or company president (or both). Care is based solely on the medical problems and what medicine has to offer.

Notwithstanding equality of care in ICUs, most physicians consider drug addicts and dealers the lowest form of life. We accept that they will lie, cheat, steal and, if necessary, kill to get what they want. But in the ICU even the lowest of the low receives the same top notch care as anyone else, even if their physical problem is 100% drug-related. Doctors and nurses often ponder the irony that the life we save today may rob us tomorrow.

So Lester's drug habit and reason for coming to MICU didn't matter. We would have done whatever necessary to salvage his brain regardless of the cause. Unfortunately there was just very little to offer the patient. Within an hour of his arrival to MICU both neurosurgery and neurology consultants confirmed the dismal prognosis.

Apart from the fact that the neurosurgeon operates, while the neurologist is mainly a diagnostician of nervous system disorders, a principal distinction between the two specialists is the amount of words they leave in a consultation note. The neurosurgeon always writes what is necessary in half a page or less. The neurologist seldom makes do with less than two pages, and sometimes writes four or five.

The neurosurgeon called to see Lester summarized the situation thus: "Massive SAH [subarachnoid hemorrhage]. Little hope for survival. Nothing to offer surgically."

The neurologist's summary was a bit longer: "In the presence of deep coma from SAH the prognosis for survival is very poor. Based on data from Levy, et al, (Annals Internal Medicine, March 1981, pages 293-301), Mr. Brown has a 74% probability of dying from this SAH. Given his specific neurologic findings, particularly absent oculocephalic response [eye movement when the head is turned] and absent corneal reflexes [blinking when the eyeball is lightly touched], Mr. Brown's chance for survival is only 5%, and even at that he would in all likelihood be in a vegetative state. I simply cannot be optimistic because of the size of his bleed and level of coma. Suggest discussion with his family regarding DNR [do not resuscitate] status. Thank you. Will follow."

Eight words vs. 116 words to say the same thing. Yet both consultants were helpful. The neurosurgeon told us that operating on the brain was of no value. The neurologist told us, authoritatively, what to expect and what to tell the family.

* * *

Lester had plenty of visitors. It was not easy to know who was related by blood and who by economic considerations. On his first day in MICU I was told he had "one brother and one sister."

The next day, two brothers and two sisters came to visit. He had no wife but at least two "girlfriends." The only relatives I felt certain about were Buba, his younger brother, and their mother, an attractive and well-dressed woman in her early 60s.

To facilitate communication everyone agreed that Buba would be the official spokesperson, and I dealt only with him. Buba was seldom alone, however; at least a few friends and relatives usually stood nearby during our conversations.

As so often happens in cases where the principle affliction is self-induced, the patient's extended family did not easily accept the drug connection. Notwithstanding Buba's comments at the time of admission, I had the distinct impression that everyone else thought something amiss happened to Lester *in* our emergency room. After all, they reasoned, Lester only came in because of a headache, albeit a severe one. "He wasn't that bad when he left home," they commented. "He was always a strong man. Healthy as an ox." Buba did little to dispel this line of thinking, either because he could not make good on his promise of retribution or because he would not admit to danger from cocaine.

As expected, Lester showed no signs of improvement. Despite full ventilator support, anti-hypertensive medication, and round-the-clock nursing, he remained deeply comatose and neurologically unresponsive.

By Lester's third day in MICU his "family" had grown to twelve people, all sitting or standing vigil in the waiting room. Although only two people are allowed in a patient's room at any one time there is no prohibiting an army, if it wishes, to camp out in the waiting area.

That afternoon I managed to catch Buba alone in Lester's room. I told him the outlook was dismal and that neither myself nor the neurologist thought Lester would survive another 24 hours. I quickly added that we would not stop the breathing machine or any other therapy, and that Lester would stay in MICU until he either died or got better. No way was I going to even hint at a slackening of care.

"Can you come out and tell that to our family? They'll want to hear it from you."

I agreed and followed Buba out to the waiting room. The four or five who were smoking (near a no-smoking sign) put away their cigarettes, and a woman on the phone hung up when she saw us coming. After everyone assembled in a corner of the large waiting area as I explained the situation.

"Unfortunately there's been no improvement in Mr. Brown's condition. The neurology specialist saw him this morning and repeated another brain wave test. It looks very bad. His brain activity is only one step above being totally brain dead. At this point, in all honesty, we don't think he's going to make it."

"You're not giving up, Doc." A command, not a question.

"Absolutely not," I retorted quickly. "I made that clear just now to Mr. Brown's brother and I promise all of you, we are in no way giving up. But Mr. Brown wanted me to tell all of you how it looks and it looks real bad."

"Well, we're going to stay right here until he gets better. Did you find out the cause yet?"

"We still think it's from cocaine," I answered matter-of-factly. "The CAT scan of his brain, the cocaine we found in his urine, and the neurologic exam all point to a ruptured blood vessel like we often see in cocaine users." I carefully refrained from using the word addict. "Sometimes this happens just from high blood pressure, but in Mr. Brown's case we think it was the cocaine." I had explained the likely chain of events several times already. This time I wanted to add, 'So all of you should quit using coke,' but didn't dare.

One of the young bucks in the crowd, either a brother or friend or business partner, looked straight at me and said, menacingly: "It ain't no cocaine that did this." I didn't respond since his comment wasn't a question.

After answering a few more questions I returned to the ICU. Silently, I hoped I would not be there when Lester died, but at the same time felt ashamed at my wish; *somebody* would have to tell the family.

*　　*　　*

Lester's blood pressure collapsed the next afternoon. I was there. In futility we pumped on his chest and infused pressor drugs but it didn't matter. His brain was gone. We pronounced him dead at 4:35.

"Are you going to tell the family?" one of the nurses asked me. She was not asking *if* I was going to tell, as if there was an option. She was asking if *I* was going to take the responsibility or delegate it to someone else.

"Sure," I said. As director of MICU what else could I say?

I looked at the intern who had assisted with the CPR, an innocent fellow named Bob. It would have been unfair to send him out alone but he had to learn to give out bad news. "Bob, why don't you come with me?" We went out together.

On the way out I whispered to Bob that the only way to do this sort of thing is to be direct. He nodded agreement. Lester's family was all very quiet as we walked toward them. I think they suspected that Lester had died and were just waiting for confirmation.

"I'm sorry," I said. "Mr. Brown just passed away."

All hell broke loose. The two girlfriends started wailing and sobbing. Lester's mother began repeating "Oh No! Oh No!" in a high pitched sing song. Then the young man who knew "it ain't no cocaine" began pounding the wall with his fist, at which point Buba tried to restrain him. This action only backfired, as the pounding man became more combative. Bob and I retreated back toward the ICU. On our way we heard "*WHAM!*" and the sound of broken plaster. The young man had broken away from Buba and put his fist through the wall. The blow would have floored Muhammad Ali in his prime.

Bob and I rushed inside MICU and called Security. I had a dead man inside and a crazy one outside. We could hear the wailing and banging continue. I feared more for innocent bystanders than for myself or the MICU staff. In fact I felt protected in MICU; they wouldn't dare enter the sanctuary of the critically ill, where Lester lay in repose.

Fortunately I was right. But outside MICU it was a different story. A minute after my call two security guards appeared. Ordinarily two guards can take care of almost any hospital disturbance but in this case they were outnumbered. The young buck's anger had infected the group so that attempts at reasoning by the guards was to no avail.

Standard policy is to escort off the hospital grounds anyone causing a disturbance. But how do you escort a dozen wailing, fist-pounding, angry people who have just lost a loved one? Well, you can't.

More security guards were called, for a total of five. A melee erupted. Punches were swung and jaws hit. Fortunately, no one had a gun or the melee would have added to our ICU census. As it turned out, one guard suffered a broken mandible and one relative had his shoulder dislocated; both were treated in the emergency room.

I saw none of the action. For an hour after the noise abated the MICU staff stayed put. Then our Chief of Security came in to report all was under control and that two officers would be stationed outside the ICU all night. Apparently one of the group had made some threatening remarks, necessitating the extra protection. There had been no arrests.

Nothing came of the threats and everything in MICU quickly returned to normal. Two hours after death was pronounced Lester's body was unceremoniously taken to the morgue.

Comment

Lester Brown was one of many cocaine victims we treat every year. Famous victims — the college basketball star Len Bias, the professional football player Don Rogers, the movie star John Belushi — are the tip of an enormous iceberg of senseless, drug-related death. At least one cocaine user is admitted to our MICU every week, for a variety of serious medical problems: coma, cerebral hemorrhage, severe hypertension, cardiac arrhythmia, pulmonary edema, pneumonia. Most patients survive their first acute medical problem but many, like Lester, do not. Of course we never see the ones who die in the street, or in a crack house.

Sudden death from cocaine is usually related to either subarachnoid hemorrhage, heart attack (coronary thrombosis) or cardiac arrhythmia. The mechanism of SAH is poorly understood but is probably due to a sudden rise in cerebral blood pressure caused by the drug, followed by rupture of a vulnerable blood vessel into the brain.

Since the case of Lester Brown several other young people have died in our MICU following a single encounter with cocaine. Anyone who uses street cocaine risks sudden death.

15. Crisis and Lysis

"Doctor Martin, I need some help." The call was from Bill Moody, a medical resident in the emergency department.

"Sure Bill, what's up?"

"There's a patient down here with severe shortness of breath and hypoxemia. He's in some distress. I think he might have a pulmonary embolism, or at least that's the only way I can put everything together. He and his wife just came back from Florida. They drove straight through, non-stop, eighteen hours in the car. I want to take him for a lung scan but wonder if I should heparinize him first."

"Don't do anything yet. I'll be right down."

Well, I thought, here it is again. Pulmonary embolism. One of the most difficult diagnoses to make and treat. The great killer, undiagnosed in half the patients who have it. Often overdiagnosed in patients who have something else. A disease that is the bane of surgeons and internists alike.

What is it? Embolus is from the Greek *embolos*, 'plug.' If a blood clot forms in a vein and travels to the lungs it causes a pulmonary embolus or embolism. A branch of the circulation within the lung captures the embolus and becomes 'plugged.' If more than one such clot travels to the lung we call them pulmonary emboli.

Pulmonary emboli may arise from veins anywhere in the body but the legs are by far the most common site of origin. Until the clots break off they are usually silent and the patient has no symptoms (although occasionally the legs swell if the clots are huge).

Once the travelling clots reach the lungs they can cause pain, shortness of breath, cough (either dry or with expectoration of blood), palpitations and a host of other symptoms. Unfortunately, given suspicion of an embolus, there is no easy way to make the diagnosis, at least with certainty. Sometimes we have to treat the patient based on inconclusive evidence. The standard therapy is intravenous heparin, a potentially dangerous blood thinner.

153

If treatment was easy pulmonary embolism wouldn't be such a big headache for doctors. Because heparin 'thins' the blood by interfering with clotting, it puts the patient at constant risk of *bleeding.* Of course heparin also prevents more clots from forming and going to the lungs, but what's the good of that if the patient has a major hemorrhage?

Another useful drug is streptokinase, but many physicians consider it even more dangerous than heparin. Either drug can improve survival from pulmonary embolism about 3-fold, but the bleeding risk from treatment mandates reasonable certainty about the diagnosis. Often the choice is between the lesser of two evils: risk of bleeding vs. risk of more (and potentially fatal) clots to the lungs.

Diagnosis is often difficult because the symptoms are non-specific. Chest pain and shortness of breath are also common symptoms in heart attack, pneumonia, pleurisy, esophagitis and many other conditions. Physicians can't treat every suspicious complaint as a pulmonary embolus, but if the diagnosis is missed that patient's next clot could be fatal.

Some people are at increased risk for pulmonary embolism: patients in a post-operative state or at prolonged bed rest or immobilization, during pregnancy, and patients with chronic heart or lung disease, or cancer. Pulmonary embolism is rare in healthy, active people, with one major exception: women taking birth control pills, especially if they smoke.

Compared to pulmonary emboli the majority of heart and lung disorders — including pneumonia, heart attack, heart failure, emphysema, and lung cancer — are relatively easy to diagnose. Pulmonary embolism is both missed *and* over diagnosed frequently. The situation is sometimes like trying to identify a relative behind an opaque glass door. If you could open the door you would have no trouble; otherwise, you can only guess who is there.

The definitive diagnostic test involves passing a catheter through the heart and into the lungs, then squirting die into the pulmonary blood vessels. This test, being invasive and expensive, is hardly routine. Instead, doctors in most hospitals rely on the lung scan, a nuclear medicine test that images the effects of the blood clots but not the clots themselves.

Unfortunately the lung scan is a very sensitive test; almost any lung condition can show up abnormal, including asthma, heart failure, emphysema, pneumonia, and so forth. Certain patterns on a lung scan favor the diagnosis of emboli. Radiologists who interpret lung scans use terms like 'high,' 'low' and 'indeterminate' to describe the probability that a given scan represents pulmonary emboli.

Of course radiologists can only interpret images as they appear on film. The clinician has to incorporate the scan interpretation into his or her own 'index of clinical suspicion.' Essentially the clinician asks: do I have a high, medium, or low suspicion that my patient has a pulmonary embolus?

When all the rigmarole is dispensed with (including opinions from several lookers-on), it comes down to something like this (PE = pulmonary embolism):

Scan Reading	Clinical Suspicion	What to do
High	High	Treat the patient
High	Low	Do another test
Indeterminate	High	Treat, or do another test
Indeterminate	Low	Abandon diagnosis of PE
Low	High	Do another test, or abandon diagnosis
Low	Low	Abandon diagnosis

It is seldom this simple but the chart gives an idea of the diagnostic process. The problem is that "another test" is either the highly invasive catheter study, or some less invasive but usually less conclusive one, such as a study to look for clots in leg veins that might (or might not) break off.

Would Dr. Moody's patient be difficult-to-diagnose or straightforward?

*   *   *

In the emergency room I met Francis Jarvin, a 50-year-old stock broker just returned from Florida with his wife, Sylvia. I was struck immediately by two things: his breathing and his suntan. Each of his breaths was deep and painful, with the pain mostly felt over his right chest. In effect he 'splinted' his breathing, checking each inspiration to minimize pain made worse by chest movement; as a result his breaths were rapid and shallow. A normal respiratory rate is 10 to 16 effortless breaths each minute; his rate was 40. Our patient wasn't shocky or confused and his vital signs were stable except for the rapid breathing.

Mr. Jarvin sported a loud Hawaii-type shirt, pink pants and white loafers, hardly the clothes we see in our Midwest patients (during February, no less). He was clean-shaven, with thinning hair and well manicured features, and sported a deep, even suntan and slight paunch. He could just as well be laying at the beach as on a hospital bed in our emergency room. The apprehension in his eyes, the too-rapid movement of his chest cage, and an oxygen mask that obscured his nose and mouth, told me he was in the right place.

About ten hours earlier, somewhere in Kentucky, Mr. Jarvin first noted chest pain and shortness of breath. He thought it might be indigestion and didn't want to stop in an unfamiliar city "if that's all it was." About an hour later his wife took over the driving. As soon as they arrived home she drove him to Memorial's emergency room. Given his level of discomfort I was amazed he'd been able to finish the trip.

The oxygen mask and breathing problem made it difficult for him to talk. I needed to be quick and direct with my examination, but also not alarm him. I asked Dr. Moody to get me his chest x-ray, blood gas report, cardiogram, and emergency room chart.

"Hi, I'm Dr. Martin. I'll be taking care of you upstairs. I just want to ask you a few questions, listen to your lungs and heart, and then you'll go for a lung scan. I understand you just came back from Florida." I spoke as if I was making conversation with an acquaintance.

"Yes...that's right."

"I know you're short of breath and in some pain. Don't try to talk. Just answer yes or no if you can, or nod your head. You drove home by car?" He nodded yes.

"You drove straight through, all twelve-hundred miles, except for stopping a few times?" Another nod.

"What's the longest you sat in the car without stopping? Just given me an approximation."

"About...five...hours...I guess." Mr. Jarvin squirmed with chest discomfort.

"Did you ever have pain in your legs?"

He shook his head.

"I understand you're taking some pills for high blood pressure."

"...Yes, my wife has them."

"Calan and Dyazide, is that right?"

He nodded agreement.

"Have you ever been in the hospital before?"

He held up one finger.

"Once?"

"Yes...for hernia...about ten years ago."

"OK. I'm not going to ask you anything else right now. Just let me check a few things."

Over the next few minutes I examined his heart, lungs, abdomen and legs, reviewed his vital signs and initial lab results, and developed a firm impression: massive pulmonary embolism.

Dr. Moody came in just as I was finishing. "They're ready for him in nuclear medicine," he said. "Should we start him on heparin?"

"No," I said. "He's going to MICU straight from the lung scan. Please call MICU and tell them we'll be there as soon as the scan's finished. Ask Marsha Ligner, the head nurse, to please order up streptokinase and have two hundred and fifty thousand units ready when we get there."

"You're going to use streptokinase?"

"If his scan shows what I think it will, that's what he needs. Heparin isn't going to help him much right now. We need to break up these clots."

I accompanied Mr. Jarvin to nuclear medicine, one floor below the emergency department. I was nervous about him. What other diagnosis could this be? I didn't know, but we needed the scan to confirm pulmonary embolism and justify using strepto-kinase. I just hoped he would finish and get to MICU before some catastrophe occurred. He seemed more unstable by the minute.

The technician injected his arm vein with the radioactive technetium, the material used for showing up the lungs, then set the scanner over his chest. I watched the images as they appeared on the monitor. In healthy lungs the radioactive material is distributed evenly throughout the open blood vessels and shows up as a pattern of fine dots with no interruptions. Blood clots in the lungs disturb the distribution of radioactivity and cause blank spaces to appear on the scan. When examined along with the patient's chest x-ray, the particular pattern of blank spaces determines the probability for pulmonary embolism.

Mr. Jarvin's scan showed enormous blank spaces, pie-shaped defects in both lungs evident from any angle the camera scanned. When all the camera angles were completed I said, "let's go." I didn't need the radiologist to tell me what I already knew. His likelihood for embolism was 'high-high.'

In another three minutes we were in MICU. It was 2:30 in the afternoon.

"Marsha, do you have the streptokinase?"

"Ready to go."

"Let's hang it."

*   *   *

Mr. Jarvin needed both streptokinase and reassurance. As the drug began flowing into his vein I explained the situation.

"You do have blood clots in your lungs," I said. "We've begun a drug that should help break them up. You'll probably continue to feel uncomfortable for a while, but you should feel better as the clots dissolve."

"I hope so," he winced.

And so did I. I thought back to Sabrina Jones, 17 years old. So young. And I was younger too, still in training and at another hospital. This high school student came in with a complaint of "chest pains," only three days after a previous hospital stay for therapeutic abortion. I remember her well: a short, obese teenager, cherubic face. She spoke with a limited vocab-ulary and, perhaps being so young, did not seem particularly apprehensive about the pains or about being *back* in the hospital so soon. She had a history of two pregnancies; the first one, just a year earlier, was brought to term. The infant boy was being cared for by Sabrina's 32-year-old mother.

The pains were sharp and fleeting, and caused her mother to bring Sabrina back to the hospital; the pains probably worried her mother more than Sabrina. Unfortunately Sabrina's legs were fat, too fat to properly examine for clots. We all thought of pulmonary embolism, considered it a possibility, and ordered the lung scan. But we didn't heparinize her right away. She was not in any distress and actually seemed comfortable on the ward. Also, just three days after a therapeutic abortion, we felt there was no point in risking bleeding until we were certain of a diagnosis. Then too, Sabrina was only 17, had no chronic diseases, and the pains could just as well have been pleurisy, a benign viral syndrome. So we ordered the scan and some pain medicine and went about our hospital rounds.

Twenty minutes later I was paged 'stat' to the nursing station; Sabrina was in sudden distress. *Acute distress*: breathing labored, nostrils flaring, neck muscles contracting, unable to speak. Her pulse raced at 140 and worse, far worse, within a minute, before our eyes, she went into shock — NO BLOOD PRESSURE! From there it was all downhill. We did CPR for one hour and 10 minutes and then called it. Sabrina was dead. From the moment I saw her in distress, I knew why.

The autopsy confirmed a massive 'saddle' embolus straddling both main branches of her pulmonary artery, completely occluding the flow of blood from heart to lungs. The pains she experienced before hospital admission were from smaller emboli, sentinels sent out to warn of impending doom. Would she have survived if treated right away with heparin? Possibly, but we'll never know. I do know that since Sabrina Jones I am sensitized to this diagnosis, respectful of what massive pulmonary embolism can do and how quickly it can snuff out a life.

* * *

I had spoken to Mrs. Jarvin only briefly in the ER and during the lung scan test. She deserved some explanation so I went out to the MICU lounge where she was sitting.

About 48 and also suntanned, with a bouffant hairdo and heavy silver earrings, Slyvia Jarvin looked tired. What a way to end a vacation, I thought. I told her of Mr. Jarvin's condition, the results of the lung scan, our use of streptokinase.

"Can he die from this?" she wanted to know right away.

I thought of Sabrina and almost blurted out 'You betcha!'

"It's possible," I said, "that's one reason he's in MICU, so we can watch him closely. We've already started streptokinase and the next few hours will be crucial. Why didn't you stop at a hospital earlier?"

"Why? Why?" she said mockingly. "Because he's bull-headed, that's why! I begged him to let me stop. He kept saying 'we'll be home in a few hours, it's just indigestion. Keep driving.' If he doesn't make it I'll never forgive myself."

"What happened when you got home?"

"He could hardly walk. He certainly couldn't lift the suitcases out of the trunk. He was sick, I knew it right away. I took one look at him and it was back in the car. We came straight here. Too bad the kids are away." The Jarvins had two grown children living elsewhere.

"Well, you did the right thing, by bringing him here as soon as possible, that's for sure."

She stayed in the MICU lounge the rest of the afternoon and visited her husband a few minutes each hour. Their suitcases remained unpacked in the car.

In the emergency department Mr. Jarvin's oxygen saturation

was 90%, a low value considering that he was inhaling extra oxygen from the face mask; normal oxygen saturation without extra oxygen is 95% or greater. In patients like Mr. Jarvin we follow both their respiratory rate and oxygen saturation, the latter with a non-invasive 'oximeter' clip that fits comfortably over the finger. A chronology of Mr. Jarvin's course that afternoon:

2:00 - Respiratory rate 40, oxygen saturation 90%
2:30 - Streptokinase begun
3:00 - RR 35, oxygen saturation 91%
4:00 - RR 31, oxygen saturation 92%
5:00 - RR 26, oxygen saturation 93%
6:00 - RR 24, oxygen saturation 94%

At 6:30 I found our patient comfortable and smiling. Sylvia was in the room. "I feel much better," he said. "I don't know what you used but it sure seems to be working."

I was glad we started streptokinase. Heparin would not have acted nearly so fast. If he didn't have a bleeding complication the prognosis was excellent.

Comment and Followup

Streptokinase was approved in 1977 for treatment of pulmonary embolism. The drug is commonly used for heart attack victims within the first four hours of symptoms, a critical period where it can open up clogged coronary vessels. Along with newer drugs of similar type, 'TPA' and 'APSAC,' streptokinase has saved lives of heart attack victims all over the world.

Streptokinase is less commonly used than heparin in PE because, in some early studies, it seemed to cause more bleeding without improving survival. Yet streptokinase breaks up the clots quicker than heparin and may *not* be any more dangerous. If used properly, and if the patient is not invaded frequently for blood drawing and other tests, the complications are about the same as with heparin. Certainly if we need to lyse a patient's blood clots quickly streptokinase (or other drugs of similar action) is the way to go. Heparin is just too slow.

We continued streptokinase infusion another 36 hours and then, according to standard protocol, switched over to intravenous heparin therapy. Mr. Jarvin stayed on heparin for several days after which he began an oral blood thinner, coumadin. There was no complication from any of the drugs and he went home on the eighth hospital day.

Mr. Jarvin took coumadin for two months, by which time he was out of the danger period. He never again subjected himself to prolonged sitting, the condition that led to venous stasis and formation of the clots.

Now he only flies to Florida.

16. Extraordinary Care

Helga Bowman was 60 when her life went into a tailspin. Within one week of March, 1982, she learned of cancer in her right breast and emphysema in both lungs.

On March 12 she consulted a surgeon for a breast lump. Suspicious right away, Dr. Spivey explained it could be cancerous and that she might need a mastectomy. He biopsied the lump with a thin needle, removing just a few cells for microscopic examination. The next day, March 13, Dr. Spivey received a verbal pathology report: malignancy. He promptly called Mrs. Bowman, told her the diagnosis, and scheduled a mastectomy for March 16. Because of her long smoking history he also ordered pulmonary function tests and asked her to see me.

Mrs. Bowman came to my office on March 14. A middle-aged, kindly-appearing woman with a big smile, she displayed all the telltale signs of emphysema: raised shoulders; slightly pursed lips; slow gait; and contraction of neck muscles with each breath. Most emphysema patients are thin and she was no exception, weighing 110 pounds and standing five feet two. She wore a plain cotton dress and little makeup, and kept her brown hair brushed straight back.

Any complaints? "I feel fine," she said, "like always. Just this lump I noticed last week." She pointed to her right breast.

"How long have you been smoking?"

"I started when I was about twenty. Forty years I guess."

"How much? Would you say a pack a day?"

"Yes, no more than that. But it never caused me any problems."

As she undressed for the exam I could see she was limited and less agile than other middle-aged woman with normal lungs. Her pattern of speech, an occasional pause to catch her breath, confirmed my visual assessment. She would look quite healthy in a family snapshot but not on videotape.

Her emphysema had developed insidiously. Shortness of breath on exertion and a chronic morning cough became such a routine experience for Mrs. Bowman that she considered the symptoms almost normal. "I thought they just happen when you get older," she explained.

Lung capacity less than 50% of normal indicates marked breathing impairment; her capacity was only 42%. This measurement, plus the chest x-ray and my examination, confirmed severe emphysema. Lung disease of this degree doesn't preclude breast surgery but does make one more cautious. Our concern is the general anesthesia, which can cause problems for patients with respiratory impairment. I insisted that Mrs. Bowman quit smoking right away, and also prescribed inhalation treatments and corticosteroids for the two remaining days before surgery.

She took the bad news and my recommendations surprisingly well. There was no denial, self-pity, or remorse sometimes seen in cancer patients. Just the opposite. The thing I remember most from her days before surgery was how *non-depressed* she seemed. Friendly and outgoing, she was the type of person who found something good in every bad situation.

On my visit to her hospital room the night before surgery I met Mr. Bowman, a 62-year-old retired fireman. Like his wife he was outgoing and affable. A short, thin man, he had the parched and wrinkled skin of an outdoorsman. Fishing was his passion. "I've spent most of my life outdoors," he said.

"What do you catch around here?" I asked him.

"Walleye. The lake's got tons of walleye this time of year. Just caught several last week."

We bantered a few minutes about the hazards of lake fishing and then I changed the subject to his wife's operation. I again discussed the risks of surgery and asked if they had any questions.

"No," they replied, with Mrs. Bowman adding, "We have faith in you and Dr. Spivey." Mr. Bowman nodded his agreement and that was that.

"By the way, you did quit smoking, didn't you?"

"Oh, yes," she said. "I'll never go back to cigarettes." The way she had accepted my no-smoking advice was a good sign. Whatever there was to do or take that might help, she would comply.

On March 16 Mrs. Bowman underwent a modified right radical

mastectomy. The operation involved removing her breast, some surrounding muscle tissue, and lymph nodes in the axillary (armpit) area that drain lymph from the breast. Several of these nodes were involved with cancer, indicating the tumor had spread outside her breast. She would need post-operative radiotherapy and chemotherapy to achieve any hope of cure.

She recovered from surgery without any problems and had an uneventful hospital course. Dr. Spivey discharged her a week later. In early April, as an outpatient, she began a regimen of 20 cobalt treatments, one each weekday. The x-ray beams were aimed to the region of her absent right breast and right shoulder area.

Two weeks later, after only 10 cobalt sessions, she developed a fever. Pus began to drain from her surgical wound. Radiation therapy was stopped and an antibiotic prescribed, but the chest wall drainage continued. A few days later we re-admitted her to the hospital.

Skin bacteria had taken hold at the site of surgery and caused a deep, bony abscess in the underlying sternum, or breast bone. Despite heavy doses of intravenous antibiotics over several days the infection continued to spread, eroding almost completely through her sternum. Unchecked, the infection might spread to her heart.

We called in a thoracic surgeon to debride the infection. The pain of deep debridement necessitated it be done under general anesthesia. Her lungs might not withstand another operation but there was little choice by this point. The infection had to be surgically removed.

At operation much of her sternum was like mush. The surgeon drained all the pus and removed several loose bone fragments, then sutured the remaining pieces of bone together with wire. The resulting assemblage of remaining sternal bone and wire did not form a solid breast plate. Although the operation effectively treated the infection, it left her with an unstable chest cage.

Mrs. Bowman was returned to MICU, still connected to the ventilator. Although her chest was covered with bandages I could see the problem. When she tried to breathe on her own, instead of the chest's normal outward movement with each breath, her chest collapsed *inward*. An unstable chest cage, added to severely weakened lungs, meant she would never be able to breathe unassisted by machine. The next day, April 10, she returned to the operating room for a tracheostomy.

Despite this major complication, and the reality that her cancer was far from cured, Mrs. Bowman remained cheerful. Metastatic breast cancer, severe emphysema, three operations, and several weeks in hospital did not daunt her spirit. She continued to have faith in her doctors and display a strong will to live, no matter what the setbacks.

At first I thought her upbeat mood was inappropriate, or at least an indication that she really didn't understand all that had happened. Certainly I would be depressed in her situation and so expected that she would be, if not clinically depressed, at least sullen, discouraged. Not her. This woman, who had two crippling diseases and a material net worth less than the yearly income of most doctors, viewed life only from the positive side. She had a good marriage, healthy children and grandchildren, and everything to live for. Why be depressed?

I did not mention that getting off the ventilator seemed unlikely (I did tell Mr. Bowman). Instead, I accented the positive. "We're going to start chemotherapy. We can't give you any more radiotherapy but the drugs should help control your tumor."

"Good," she said with her lips. The tracheostomy tube prevented speech but her facial expression said, 'let's get on with it so I can get better and go home'.

Over the next month we gave her the latest in cancer chemotherapy. She developed complications, first pneumonia, then urinary tract infection, then a stormy course of high fever and sepsis. At one point we thought she would not survive, but her body rallied and the infections were brought under control. She remained cheerful. The same could not be said for her doctors.

The oncologist and radiotherapist decided that she could receive no more cancer therapy and signed off her case. There was no evidence of tumor recurrence, but her fragile state made it impossible to give additional treatments if the tumor did recur.

At the end of a month in MICU, after her recovery from sepsis, I again tried to wean her off the ventilator. As expected, the effort was unsuccessful. Her lungs and chest wall were all but destroyed. Thus it came to be that, two months after the initial diagnosis of breast cancer, Mrs. Bowman lay in a MICU bed as a pure "pulmonary" case — and a disposition dilemma. Where could we send a 60-year-old, ventilator-dependent woman?

Ordinarily we would have looked for one of the rare nursing homes that accept ventilator patients. She would not consider it. Neither she nor her husband wanted her to be in a nursing home. Mr. Bowman had the solution.

"I'll take her home with me."

Before Mrs. Bowman's case, all of Memorial Medical Center's ventilator-dependent patients either died in the hospital or went to a nursing home. I knew that other hospitals had sent one or two ventilator-dependent cases home, but those patients were wealthy. The Bowmans barely made ends meet on Mr. Bowman's modest pension.

Artificial ventilation at home requires an oxygen supply company able to manage the ventilator and someone to care for the patient round the clock. The first requirement is easy, since third party payers will cover the ventilator care at home (it is cheaper than in a hospital). The second requirement is the usual stumbling block. Continuous nursing care is prohibitively expensive and insurance companies will not pay for it. Family members can theoretically do the job, but who has family that can dedicate to such extraordinary care? As it turned out, Mrs. Bowman did: Mr. Bowman.

I had my doubts. Mr. Bowman was devoted to his wife, but could he alone do the tasks that, in the hospital, require several shifts of workers? We would not discharge Mrs. Bowman until she was stable, but even then she would require almost constant attention. She needed to be suctioned often, given a bed pan when necessary, and fed three meals a day; the ventilator had to be checked instantly if any alarms went off; and calls had to be made if something went wrong.

Yes, yes, yes, Mr. Bowman insisted. He could do whatever was needed. All we had to do was show him what and how. Having no reasonable alternative, we agreed to send Mrs. Bowman home with a ventilator.

It took about a week for the oxygen supply company to set up a ventilator in their home. To make things easier we insisted on the same model used in the hospital. The company first surveyed the house and decided the only place for the machine was a tiny first floor den. It could not go into their larger second floor bedroom because the connecting oxygen tanks were too heavy for any area but the basement. To properly connect the ventilator to the oxygen tanks required that the machine be located on the first floor. (Hospitals use a built-in liquid oxygen system with outlets in every patient room.)

After two weeks of discharge planning, during which Mr. Bowman received instruction from therapists and nurses, Mrs. Bowman was ready to leave the hospital. On the trip from MICU to the emergency room, where the ambulance was waiting to transport her home, a respiratory therapist breathed her lungs manually, with an AMBU bag. In the ambulance she received ventilation from a portable, battery-operated ventilator. Besides the two ambulance attendants, a nurse and respiratory therapist also came with her. Mr. Bowman followed the ambulance in his car and I followed in my car. I also took along our head of Respiratory Therapy; this was a first for him as well.

I had never been to her neighborhood and knew only that it was in a blue collar district about five miles south of the hospital. We followed Mr. Bowman off an expressway exit that I had passed many times before. Less than 500 feet from the exit the ambulance stopped in front of an aging, two-story wood frame house. Across the street was a gas station and a bar.

She lived on the fringe of a poor working-class section of town, in a house that was modest even by neighborhood standards. On the lot next door a rusting 1960s Ford rested on cinder blocks, its wheels and one door missing. Adjacent to the gas station was a vacant lot packed with 10 partly-stripped cars. In the air, the din of the expressway with high-decibel trucks roaring by every few minutes, and a pervasive smell of exhaust fumes. Though not a slum, the neighborhood was far from appealing. I looked around and thought: *this* is where we are sending our first home-ventilator patient?

As for the Bowmans, they were glad to be home. Mr. Bowman made no apologies for the place, either direct or implied. "Come on in," he welcomed with enthusiasm.

The attendants took Mrs. Bowman out of the ambulance on a stretcher and, while the nurse bagged her manually, carried her up two concrete steps and into the house. Mr. Bowman directed everyone to her new bedroom, a linoleum-floored space approximately 12 feet square. Its walls were covered with musty, stained panelling and a single window looked out on the freeway exit (in the distance I could see a large green overhead sign pointing the way to 'Downtown'). In one corner of the room was her bed, really a cot. Next to the cot stood a Puritan Bennett model MA-1 volume ventilator, its hoses arched in the air, ready for connection. What an incongruous sight!

We moved Mrs. Bowman from the stretcher to the bed and connected her to the ventilator. Mr. Bowman fussed with her a little, fixing her pillow and a blanket, while we checked her tracheostomy tube and then connected the ventilator. I turned the machine on. Whoosh! Whoosh! It worked fine. All the alarms were checked. While the therapists gave Mr. Bowman a final review of the machine's functions I briefly examined our patient. Her vital signs were OK and she was comfortable in her 'new' quarters. Careful planning had made the transition go quite smoothly.

The plan was to have the oxygen company's respiratory therapists visit the house twice a week, and for them to call me with any medical questions or special problems. Mr. Bowman planned to be home all the time; he would call for help as needed. On occasion their daughter might be able to help out, but responsibility for round-the-clock care clearly rested with Mr. Bowman.

Before leaving the house I walked around to see the other rooms. All were small, musty, and worn. The dwelling was not dirty; the kitchen, in particular, seemed clean, but I remember feeling depressed about the place and wondering why. Every room, apart from being tiny and cluttered (an ironing board, old TV, fishing equipment, and cardboard boxes filled with magazines

occupied half the living room), had that worn-out-linoleum look.
No matter how hard you cleaned this house it would always seem
tired and old. Was this place a proper abode for a ventilator-
dependent patient?

A half hour after we arrived Mrs. Bowman was safely in her
bed and stabilized. After making sure everything checked out we
said goodby and left. Outside, I looked at our chief therapist and
he looked at me. We each had the same thought.

"Not very comfortable quarters, is it?" he said.

"No, her room at the hospital was bigger."

"Well, her husband's really devoted. He's learned everything
we can teach him about the ventilator."

"It's amazing," I said. "You hear some homeowners complain
about their crabgrass, or problems with the swimming pool, or
their need for a hot water tub. The Bowmans don't have a pot to
piss in and he brings her home on a ventilator!"

The external appearance of the house, the freeway-exit
location, the size of the rooms, and the interior decor all made
for a very depressing dwelling. But Mr. Bowman was not
depressed, nor was his wife, the woman with cancer and
emphysema. *We* were depressed. How long could she live under
these circumstances? In this house?

*   *   *

During two months in the hospital, almost all spent connected
to a ventilator, Mrs. Bowman had suffered innumerable invasions
of her artery for a sample of blood. We needed the blood to
check oxygen and carbon dioxide levels and thereby adjust
ventilator settings. I had never cared for any viable patient on a
ventilator without obtaining at least one arterial blood sample a
day.

We had also ordered numerous chest x-rays (once a day while
she was in MICU) and many other tests, even when she was
stable and only waiting to be discharged.

I did not know how often we would do *any* tests now that she
was home. I didn't even know when I would get to see her again.
The oxygen company took good care of the machine, and their

technician called me once a week to report on her progress. "She's doing well," he said. "No problems with the ventilator. Mr. Bowman is managing things better than we expected. We just go in and do the maintenance checks." Given her benign course, I saw no compelling reason to make a house visit anytime soon.

About a month after she left the hospital I got a call from her husband. "Her tracheostomy cuff is leaking. I think it needs to be changed." The cuff is a small inflatable balloon at the end of the tracheostomy tube; it is normally inflated with air to provide a seal inside the trachea. If the cuff leaks and deflates, the ventilator cannot deliver the proper amount of air to the lungs.

"Is she getting enough air?" I asked.

"Yes, right now she is. But I have to keep inflating the cuff about every hour or the ventilator alarm goes off." Changing her tracheostomy tube was the one thing Mr. Bowman did not feel comfortable doing. It required disconnecting the ventilator for a minute, and that made him anxious.

"OK. I'll be out this afternoon," I said, and made plans to stop on my way home. Her house was out of the way but I didn't mind. I welcomed the opportunity to help Mr. Bowman, even with a small service. I arrived about 6 p.m. and found that her tracheostomy cuff was indeed leaking. I had brought two spares and used one as a replacement.

Mrs. Bowman was all smiles when she saw me. After I changed the tube she wrote on her pad: "Thank you."

"Are you having any problems?" I asked. "Anything bothering you? "No," she wrote. "I feel good." My examination showed that she was about the same as when she left the hospital.

Outside in the yard, where Mr. Bowman preferred to talk, I asked him, "How are you managing?"

"Just fine. I sure am glad you came out. That's real nice of you."

"No problem," I said. "Glad to do it. She seems to be holding up pretty well. Have you been out of the house since we brought her home?"

"No, our daughter does the shopping and I just stay here and take care of Helga."

"Can you do this all by yourself?"

"Sure. Maggie [their daughter] helps with the cooking sometimes, but I'm a darn good cook too. We do OK."

'Amazing', I thought, this man deserves some kind of medal!

Two months went by before I got another call. Same problem. Well, I thought, that seems about right. These trach cuffs last only about two months even in the hospital. I went out to the house and changed her tracheostomy tube.

By my exam she seemed to be doing well. There were no bedsores that you often see in nursing home patients and her spirit remained remarkably good. Mr. Bowman was taking good care of his wife. I had thought of bringing a syringe and drawing some blood samples but decided against it. Four months had passed and nothing untoward had happened. What would I do with the results?

Outside I asked Mr. Bowman, "Have you been able to get away yet?"

"I've been to the store a couple of times. Maggie stay's with her then, but its only for a short time."

"Can't you get away more often?" I was concerned about him.

"No. Maggie's got two kids of her own to care for. I'm doing fine," he said. "Don't worry about me. I don't mind staying home."

I decided not to push it.

*   *   *

Over the next two years I made another eight house calls, all to change her tracheostomy tube. I always found her cheerful and appreciative of my visits. She was never out of bed when I came, although I knew she did sit in a chair on those occasions when Mr. Bowman lifted her out. As for her husband, except for an occasional foray to the store he did not leave the house. He had not gone fishing since we brought Mrs. Bowman home from the hospital.

During those first two years Mrs. Bowman did not have a single blood test or chest x-ray. Word began to spread through the hospital of this indomitable woman at home on the ventilator, in whom not a single blood gas had been drawn in two years. I gave all the credit to the patient and her husband.

One day in August 1984 Mr. Bowman called. "She's got some pain and can't see out of one eye," he said. She had become suddenly blind in her right eye and his description made me suspect a detached retina.

"Call the ambulance," I said. "She needs to be seen by an ophthalmologist."

Two years and two months after she left Memorial Hospital she came back to our MICU. An eye surgeon saw her right away, diagnosed a detached retina and recommended surgery the next morning. It would have to be done under general anesthesia.

To prepare Mrs. Bowman for eye surgery I did an arterial blood gas and other routine tests. All the results were normal or unchanged from 1982. The operation was a success and she went home a week later, her vision improved.

*   *   *

I followed Mrs. Bowman at home for three more years. During this period I changed her tracheostomy tube about every two to four months. (I always waited for Mr. Bowman's call and always came the same day. I was out of town once and then my partner went to the house). In those three years she had no blood tests or chest x-rays.

One day in June 1987 Mr. Bowman called. "Doc, she's not doing well. Her feet and belly are swollen and she's falling asleep all the time."

"How long has this been going on?"

"Oh, about a week."

"Does she complain about anything? Any pain or difficulty breathing?"

"No, she just looks bad, Doc, real bad."

"I'll be right out."

I feared the worst, but took some diuretic and heart medicine with me in case her problem was a simple case of congestive heart failure. Maybe I could treat her at home and keep her more comfortable than she would be in a sterile hospital bed.

Pulling up to the house I mentally noted the scene: not much different from five years earlier, except that the lot filled with junk cars was now vacant and the Ford on cinder blocks was gone. The expressway hummed as before and the Bowman's house appeared about five years more decrepit.

Mr. Bowman greeted me just as I got out of the car. He repeated his earlier observation. "Thanks for coming, Doc. She looks bad, real bad."

I went to the room and found her very lethargic. I shook her gently and raised my voice: "Mrs. Bowman! Mrs. Bowman!" She smiled and acknowledged my presence but the old cheeriness was no longer there. Both feet were engorged with edema fluid but I quickly discerned a different reason for the abdominal swelling. Her liver was rock hard, the first indication after five years that the breast cancer had spread. I went outside to talk to Mr. Bowman.

"I'm suspicious that her cancer has come back," I said.

"I was afraid of that."

"There's little we can do if that's the case. She's had all the therapy possible and there's nothing else to offer."

"Can she go to the hospital and die there? The grandchildren are always coming over and..." He started to cry. I fought the same urge.

"Sure," I said. "Just wait here. I'll take care of it. Let me make a phone call."

I went to the kitchen to use the phone. After making the arrangements I returned to Mr. Bowman, who was still outside the house.

"The ambulance will be here in a few minutes. I've also phoned the hospital. We'll have a bed for her in the intensive care unit."

"Thanks, Doc." He was still crying.

Followup

Our tests confirmed that the breast cancer had recurred and spread to her liver. We kept Mrs. Bowman in MICU for two days and then transferred her to a regular ward, where she received routine ventilator and nursing care. We kept her comfortable with morphine injections. Mrs. Bowman died in her sleep a week later.

As for Mr. Bowman, he still lives in the same house, alone, although his grandchildren visit often. And after a five year hiatus he is back fishing regularly for walleye.

17. Thyroid Storm

I'll never forget the patient Roberta Smith, a 35-year-old mother of two who presented to our emergency department with fever, confusion and a very fast heart beat. After a brief evaluation in the ED she was sent to MICU.

As they rolled Mrs. Smith into MICU on a stretcher I could *see* her problem. Set inside a thin face of smooth and shiny complexion were eyes that bulged like a frog's. A large mass straddled her windpipe and neck veins on either side pulsated rapidly with the rhythm of her heart. She manifested the classic picture of an extremely overactive thyroid gland, so extreme as to deserve the appellation 'thyroid storm.'

I examined the ED ledger and x-rays while the nurses put her to bed. The admitting diagnosis was actually pneumonia, with "possible hyperthyroidism" a secondary diagnosis. On chest x-ray her pneumonia showed up as a hazy infiltrate in one lung.

There is no test comparable to an x-ray for diagnosing hyperthyroidism, which is why the ED doctor hedged his diagnosis. Laboratory confirmation is based on blood tests that take much longer to process than any x-ray. Since hyperthyroidism is rarely life-threatening, doctors always wait for blood results if the patient is not acutely ill. In cases where the diagnosis seems apparent *and* the patient is toxic, treatment is begun immediately.

I asked Mrs. Smith a few questions but she did not answer. Instead she just stared at me with eyes bursting out of their sockets and moaned: *"Ummmmmmmmmmmmmmmmmmmmmm. Ummmmmmmmmmmmmm."*

How had this woman gone untreated for so long?

* * *

The thyroid gland straddles the trachea or windpipe. Although the gland is normally not visible, it can be felt in some people as a slight bulge in the neck area. Mrs. Smith's thyroid gland was at least triple normal size and easy to see. Size alone doesn't indicate overactivity; some of the largest thyroid glands, or goiters as they are called, are inactive. Mrs. Smith's gland was both big and overactive.

Thyroid hormone regulates the body's metabolism. When there is too little hormone the patient is 'hypothyroid.' Hypothyroid patients frequently complain of feeling sluggish, intolerant of cold and fatigued. Hyperthyroid patients — those with too much thyroid hormone — are often nervous, jittery and tachycardic. The most extreme cases of thyroid imbalance, high or low, represent a medical emergency.

The clinical exam of Mrs. Smith reads like a textbook case of hyperthyroidism:

Skin warm and moist.
Temperature 102 degrees.
Pounding heart, rate 150 per minute.
Wide, bulging eyes showing twice as much white sclera as
     normal (medical term: exophthalmos)
Large thyroid gland
Muscle weakness in all extremities
Muscle reflexes 4+ (hyperactive)
Fine tremor in both hands
Intolerant of heat (does not keep bed covers on)
Displays emotional lability, ranging in a span of 20 minutes
     from an unresponsive, moaning state to smiling euphoria
     to crying to laying quiet.

Mrs. Smith's medical diagnosis was Graves' disease*, a disorder of altered immunology that allows thyroid hormone to pour out unchecked by normal feedback mechanisms. As is often the case with acutely thyrotoxic patients, she had probably suffered 'smoldering hyperthyroidism' from Graves' disease for many

---

* Since the disease is named after Robert Graves, the grammatically correct spelling should be Graves's disease. However, almost all modern medical texts, as well as unabridged dictionaries, spell it Graves' disease.

months. Pneumonia then pushed her over the brink and into a state of severe thyrotoxicosis (thyroid storm).

Graves' disease is an "autoimmune" phenomenon, which means the patient's own antibodies attack some portion of the thyroid gland, altering the normal regulation of thyroid hormone production. This may be the mechanism but it does not explain the basic cause (why do some people generate antibodies to their own thyroid?), which remains unknown. Stress was once thought to play a role but this has never been substantiated.

Graves' disease afflicts an estimated one million Americans every year, with women contracting the disease much more commonly than men. Usually the patient with Graves' hyperthyroidism has a benign course and can be treated as an *outpatient*. What made Mrs. Smith's hyperthyroidism so special was its *rapid and severe* presentation.

(In the spring of 1991 President Bush developed a cardiac arrhythmia — atrial fibrillation — from previously undiagnosed Graves' disease. Two years earlier Mrs. Bush also was diagnosed with Graves' disease. Familial association, i.e. Graves' disease among blood relatives, has been long known but occurrence in spouses is rare; as far as anyone knows the disease is not 'catching' or communicable. In any event their hyperthyroidism was a much milder form than that seen in thyroid storm.)

*   *   *

Robert James Graves was an Irish physician who lived from 1795 to 1853. He is known mainly for his classic paper on hyperthyroidism, published in the London Medical and Surgical Journal in 1835; a portion of this paper is quoted below. (From Ralph H. Major, M.D., *Classic Descriptions of Disease*, 3rd Edition, 1945. Courtesy of Charles C. Thomas, Publisher, Springfield, Illinois.)

NEWLY OBSERVED AFFECTION OF THE THYROID GLAND IN FEMALES
I have lately seen three cases of violent and long continued palpitations in females, in each of which the sample

peculiarity presented itself, viz. enlargement of the thyroid gland, at all times considerably greater than natural, was subject to remarkable variations in every one of these patients. When the palpitations were violent the gland used notably to swell and become distended, having all the appearance of being increased in size in consequence of an interstitial and sudden effusion of fluid into its substance...

A lady, aged twenty, became affected with some symptoms, which were supposed to be hysterical. This occurred more than two years ago; her health previously had been good. After she had been in this nervous state about three months it was observed that her pulse had become singularly rapid. This rapidity existed without any apparent cause and was constant, the pulse being never under 120, and often much higher. She next complained of weakness on exertion, and began to look pale and thin. Thus she continued for a year, but during this time she manifestly lost ground on the whole, the rapidity of the heart's action having never ceased. It was now observed that the eyes assumed a singular appearance, for the eyeballs were apparently enlarged, so that when she slept or tried to shut her eyes the lids were incapable of closing. When the eyes were open, the white sclerotic could be seen, to a breadth of several lines, all around the cornea...

*   *   *

The account by Graves was soon followed by that of Carl A. von Basedow, a German contemporary. Basedow's article appeared in a German medical journal March 28, 1840, part of which is quoted below. (From Ralph H. Major, M.D., *Classic Descriptions of Disease*, 3rd Edition, 1945. Courtesy of Charles C. Thomas, Publisher, Springfield, Illinois.)

Madame F., brunette, well built, of a decided phlegmatic temperament [married and had four children]. Madame F. felt herself very exhausted, suffered from an obstinate diarrhoea, had night sweats, lost a great deal of weight; at which time the eyeballs began to protrude from the *Orbita*. The patient complained of shortness of breath; she had a very rapid, small pulse; a resounding heart beat, she could not hold her hand still, spoke with a striking rapidity; and she liked to seat herself (because she always felt burning hot) with naked breasts and arms, in a cold draft. She showed unnatural excitement and carelessness about her condition. She went around a great deal, without being at all disturbed about her striking appearance in company. She satisfied without any afterthoughts her various strong appetites, slept well, however with open eyes.

Sometime in 1837 however, all of these symptoms increased in intensity...in the neck there appeared a strumous swelling of the thyroid gland; the area of pulsation of the heart was now broadened, pointing to enlargement ...the hastiness of speech and the unnatural excitement of the patient still more increased, night sweats, very offensive; urine scanty and read and, considering the continued diarrhoea, the appetite was always too strong. As far as the eyes were concerned, they were pushed out so far that one could see below and above the Cornea...the eyelids were pushed wide from one another; could not be closed with every effort. The patient slept with eyes entirely open.

...For a long time, the rumor was widespread in our town that this patient was crazy and was soon going to be taken to an asylum, and in fact she had an unfriendly attitude towards the physician; she never had, however, and that I can assure you, any insane ideas; she never showed any abnormal desires and if her astonishing carelessness over her truly sad condition seemed to be the result of her phlegmatic temperament, so the hastiness of her speech, the uncertain holding of her body and her hands, the tendency to go about naked or very lightly dressed, were undoubtedly symptoms of her heart disease.

Graves did not describe any treatment for his three patients. Basedow, for his well-built brunette, first administered leeches, then "spring waters" with "marked improvement." Based on modern understanding of hyperthyroidism, *no* 19th century therapy could have been expected to benefit the patient.

For decades after their original accounts hyperthyroidism was

known as *both* Graves' and Basedow's disease.   In the first
edition of his comprehensive textbook of medicine, published in
this country in 1892, William Osler wrote:

> EXOPHTHALMIC GOITRE (GRAVES'S DISEASE;
> BASEDOW'S DISEASE).
>
> *Definition.* A disease of unknown origin, characterized by
> exophthalmos, enlargement of the thyroid, and functional
> disturbance of the vascular system...The disease is rare in
> men. Worry, fright, and depressing emotions preceded the
> development of the disease in a number of cases.
>
> *Symptoms.* In the acute form the disease may develop with
> great rapidity. In a patient of J.H. Lloyd's, of Philadelphia,
> a woman, aged thirty-nine, who had been considered
> perfectly healthy, but whose friends had noticed that for
> some time her eyes looked rather prominent, was suddenly
> seized with intensive vomiting and diarrhoea, rapid action of
> the heart and great throbbing of the arteries. The eyes
> were prominent and staring and the thyroid gland was found
> much enlarged and soft. The gastro-intestinal symptoms
> continued, the pulse became more rapid, the vomiting was
> incessant, and the patient died on the third day of the
> illness.
>
> *Treatment.* Medicinal measures are notoriously uncertain...
> Treatment of the thyroid gland itself is rarely successful,
> and the operative measures have not been very satisfactory.

In the United States today the disease described by Osler is
known only as Graves' disease. In Europe 'Basedow's disease' is
the preferred eponym.

The first effective treatment for any cause of hyperthyroidism
was surgical removal of the gland, an operation called thyroidectomy. Although it was not very successful in Osler's time, by
the 1920s, with better control of infection and bleeding,
thyroidectomy was accepted treatment for large goiters, including
those associated with hyperthyroidism.

The first effective drug therapy was inorganic iodine, a method first reported in 1923. In small amounts inorganic iodine stimulates thyroid production but in large amounts it causes the opposite effect — a lowering of thyroid hormone. Initially, inorganic iodine was used only to prepare patients for thyroidectomy; the operation is less risky if the patient's thyroid gland is first put to rest.

In the 1940s both specific anti-thyroid drugs and radioactive iodine were introduced (RAI), making it possible to treat hyperthyroidism *without* surgery. One of the specific anti-thyroid drugs, propylthiouracil or PTU, is still widely used today.

Although PTU and inorganic iodine block overactive thyroid function, they are not definitive treatment. If the patient stops the medication hyperthyroid symptoms usually recur. To permanently treat hyperthyroidism the gland must be ablated. Ablation can be accomplished either surgically or by radioactive iodine (RAI).

RAI comes as a liquid preparation that is swallowed by the patient. The radioactive iodine enters the blood and is taken up by the thyroid gland, where it destroys active thyroid cells. As a result, the gland shrinks in size. Most patients who take RAI ultimately become *hypo*thyroid within a few years. Fortunately *hypo*thyroidism is easier to treat than *hyper*thyroidism, so RAI remains an accepted and well tolerated therapy.

In summary, there are three different methods for treating hyperthyroidism: long-term anti-thyroid medication (such as PTU); RAI (a liquid that is swallowed once); and surgery. Each therapy has good and bad features. Generally, radioactive iodine (RAI) is avoided in women of child-bearing years. Surgery is preferred if the patient is non-compliant with taking medication. In middle-aged, compliant patients, either RAI or anti-thyroid medication is preferred. (Both President and Mrs. Bush received RAI therapy.)

Ultimately the decision as to which type of therapy is based on the patient's particular circumstances and the experience of the treating physician.

*   *   *

I reviewed Mrs. Smith's case with Dr. Joel Stanley, one of the MICU interns.

"Joel, have you ever seen this before?" I asked, referring to her thyroid disease.

"Graves' disease? I've seen Graves' disease, but nothing like her."

"They started penicillin in the ED," I noted. "That's probably OK for her pneumonia. They also drew all the necessary thyroid function tests. We'll get those results in a couple of days but we have to treat the hyperthyroidism now. What do you want to give her?"

He pulled out his spiral-bound book of intensive care therapy. "Let's see. They recommend several possible treatments."

"By the time you read that book she could be much worse," I replied in a friendly manner. He was certainly right to research the proper therapy but she needed treatment right away.

"Joel, while you're reading, let's give her one milligram of intravenous propranolol."

"They mention propranolol," he said, pointing to a paragraph in his book.

"Good. I hope so. It's probably the best thing to use initially in thyroid storm. Propranolol doesn't treat the hyperthyroid gland directly, but it'll slow down her heart. Then we can work on the thyroid gland itself.

Mrs. Smith's heart was in danger of failing from too rapid a rate. Propranolol, a popular cardiac drug also known as Inderal, is excellent for modulating an extremely fast heart beat.

"What do you want to give next?" I asked him.

"The next step should be an anti-thyroid drug."

"Right. Let's start propylthiouracil, two hundred milligrams every four hours. We'll have to put it down a nasogastric tube. I don't think she can take anything by mouth right now. What else besides PTU?"

"Well," he said, "I suppose we ought to add some inorganic iodine."

"Good idea," I said. "Let's start potassium iodide. Put five drops in some orange juice and put it down her NG tube every six hours."

Iodine is part of thyroid hormone. Giving the drug in its inorganic form helps block thyroid hormone release from the gland. Since inorganic iodine works more quickly than any other anti-thyroid drug we usually give it to the sickest patients, starting about one hour after the PTU.

After we began Mrs. Smith's treatment I went out to look for her family. No one was around. Apparently her husband had left the emergency department as soon as she was transferred to MICU. The phone number listed on the ED sheet went unanswered.

Two hours later Mr. Smith showed up at the hospital again. I explained his wife's condition, and told him she was receiving treatment for both pneumonia and hyperthyroidism.

"How did she get like this?" I asked.

"What do you mean?" he asked innocently.

"Well, hyperthyroidism rarely comes on all of a sudden, without any warning. How long has she been so sick?"

"I don't know," he confessed. "She hasn't been feeling well for a while. She's had some diarrhea and headaches for about a week, but we just thought it was the flu. She made an appointment to see a doctor, but that was for next week. Then last night she started coughing and running high fever. She felt no better this morning so I brought her here right away."

"Have you noticed her eyes getting more prominent?" I asked.

"Well, yes, now that you mention it. But only in the last couple of weeks."

"So what happened today?"

"This morning she couldn't get out of bed to help our older kid get ready for school. She said she didn't feel well. I got him off to school and then went to check on her. She started acting like she didn't know me, and that's when I noticed that funny stare in her eyes. I got scared and just picked her up and brought her here."

"What did the doctors say downstairs?"

"They talked to me for a few minutes and said her problem was pneumonia and maybe an overactive thyroid gland, just like you said, and that she had to go to intensive care. They said she'd be OK but she had to be watched very closely. I still had the baby with me, so I left to take her to the sitter's, where she is now. Then I came back."

"Has your wife ever had a thyroid problem before?"

"No, not as far as I know. But she has been kind of high strung for the past year. She saw a doctor about six months ago and he gave her some Valium, but we never knew it might be from this thyroid gland. At least he never said anything about it."

*   *   *

By the next morning Mrs. Smith was much improved. Her pulse was down to 110 a minute and she was coherent. A followup chest x-ray showed clearing of her pneumonia, so penicillin seemed to be the right antibiotic. In another 24 hours she was able to leave MICU.

Followup

Mrs. Smith's pneumonia continued to improve and she stayed in the hospital only three more days. Blood tests drawn on the day of admission confirmed a markedly over-active thyroid gland. Potassium iodide was discontinued at the time of discharge. For the next several months she took only PTU for her thyroid disorder.

Despite PTU she continued to experience intermittent symptoms from hyperthyroidism. After six months of PTU her endocrinologist decided to administer radioactive iodine (she planned to have no more children). As expected, the RAI obliterated most of her thyroid gland and she became *hypo*thyroid several months later. Thyroid hormone replacement was started as soon as her gland's output fell below normal. She never suffered symptoms of hypothyroidism.

Mrs. Smith now takes synthetic thyroid hormone, one pill a day. Her eyes have decreased in size considerably but are still somewhat prominent. Most importantly, she is satisfied with her appearance and feels completely well.

18. From ARC to AIDS

"Now that he's waking up don't you think somebody should tell him he has AIDS?" said Monica, one of the MICU nurses.

"He doesn't have AIDS," I responded.

"Well, somebody should tell him he is antibody positive," she said. "He could have AIDS, couldn't he?"

The patient in question was Graham Riley, a 36-year-old drug addict recovering from severe pneumonia. We ordered an HIV antibody test the day he arrived in MICU. The positive result had just returned and it was generating a lot of discussion on rounds. No one was surprised that he was HIV positive; a large number of our drug addicts were testing antibody positive in 1987. The concern at the time was: 'did he have AIDS?' By strict criteria he did not, but I sensed some confusion among the staff.

Nurses have legitimate anxieties about patients like Mr. Riley. For one thing, nurses have more hands-on contact with such patients than other health care workers, including physicians. Although all drug addicts are treated as if they harbor blood-transmissible diseases, AIDS is a special case, understandably more feared than hepatitis. Also, nurses spend more time in the room talking to patients and are apt to be asked a lot of questions. Nurses want to be able to answer them.

I addressed Kevin Edwards, the intern taking care of Mr. Riley. "Kevin, what's Mr. Riley's status this morning?"

"He's more alert today, Dr. Martin. He knows who and where he is, and the year."

"Well," I said, "that's quite an improvement." For the past week Mr. Riley had been too ill and confused to know anything, a result of both cocaine overdose and pneumonia. After six days in MICU he was responding to antibiotics and on his way to complete recovery.

"Have you told him anything about the HIV test yet?"

"No, not yet," said Kevin. "I just got the result back early this morning."

"When do you plan to tell him?"

"When he's fully alert, I guess."

"I agree, but *what* will you tell him?"

"That his antibody test for the AIDS virus is positive, but that it doesn't mean he *has* AIDS. That so far he doesn't meet the criteria for acquired immunodeficiency syndrome."

"What about ARC? Does everyone know what ARC is?"

"Well, I must admit I'm now confused," said Monica.

"Me too," replied another nurse.

"Kevin, why don't you explain ARC versus AIDS."

"OK. ARC stands for AIDS-Related Complex. It's a non-specific illness that some people get when they first become infected with the AIDS virus. It's like a bad case of the flu caused by the AIDS virus.

"But ARC is not AIDS," I added.

"Right. ARC is not AIDS and doesn't mean that AIDS will develop any time soon. In fact, most people who develop AIDS give no history of a preceding illness like ARC.

"OK," I said, "but just what constitutes ARC?"

"ARC consists of lymphadenopathy [swollen lymph nodes], weight loss, and a positive antibody to HIV [human immunodeficiency virus, the cause of AIDS]. Sometimes people with ARC also have diarrhea and low grade fever."

"Why isn't that AIDS?" asked Monica.

"The definition of AIDS requires that patients be immune compromised *and* have an opportunistic infection. We don't have any evidence for such an infection in Mr. Riley."

What Kevin said was perfectly true but needed a little amplification.

"Mr. Riley's lymphocytes are normal, something you don't see in AIDS," I said. "Based on the lymphocyte test he is not immune compromised. More importantly, the cause of his pneumonia is not an opportunistic-type organism that you see in AIDS, but is instead ordinary bacteria. If we found *pneumocystis carinii* in his lungs, then he would have *pneumocystis carinii* pneumonia and meet the criteria for AIDS. PCP is an opportunistic infection caused by a protozoa; non-immuno-compromised people don't develop PCP.

"Now as far as we know Mr. Riley does not have any opportunistic infection. His pneumonia is from *streptococcus*, the type of infection any of us could get. Also, he is responding to penicillin, a drug that doesn't work in AIDS infections.

"He does have adenopathy and has been losing weight," I continued. "Given the fact that he is HIV positive, it looks like he has the AIDS-Related Complex. He probably developed ARC a few weeks ago, and on top of that got bacterial pneumonia. Any IV drug abuser is at increased risk for ordinary pneumonia. I know the distinction between ARC and AIDS may seem confusing but it is important."

"No, I understand now," said Monica. "But what are his chances of actually getting AIDS?"

"Well, pretty good, since probably everyone with HIV antibody will develop AIDS sooner or later. Probably on the order of 20% a year for the next five years, unless some drug is developed to prevent it. But ARC itself usually improves spontaneously and does not lead directly to AIDS. Several years may elapse between ARC and the development of actual AIDS. If he continues to recover from pneumonia and his ARC remits, he'll feel healthy again."

"How are you going to explain all that to him?" asked Jennie, MICU's social worker.

"I thought I'd leave that up to you, Jennie."

She laughed. Jennie was so involved in discussing difficult social problems with our patients — and so good at it — that explaining ARC vs AIDS to a patient would have posed no big hurdle.

"Just kidding, Jennie, just kidding. It's Kevin's job. Kevin, how are *you* going to explain this? First of all, *should* we bother explaining it to him?"

"Aren't you obligated to?" asked Monica again.

"What does everyone think?"

The general consensus was yes, that if you do the test you should explain the result and provide proper counselling. No argument there.

"I'll tell him his antibody test is positive," said Kevin, "but that we don't think he has AIDS. I'll tell him that some of his symptoms are probably related to the AIDS virus, but that a positive antibody result is not the same thing as AIDS."

"Are you going to send him for counselling?" asked Jennie. "We are starting up an AIDS counselling clinic next month, and you could give him an appointment.

"Absolutely we'll give him an appointment," I said. "But he needs drug counselling more than anything. Chances are he could die of bacterial endocarditis [severe heart infection] from IV drugs well before he dies of AIDS.

"Anyway, if Kevin spends some time with him and lets him ask questions, that should help begin the educational process. The reason I want to discuss this now, outside his room, is that I don't want a hoard of people going in to confront him with the HIV result. Too many people will just inhibit any discussion. It's best if Kevin and maybe you, Monica, go in later today or tomorrow, when he's fully alert."

"Good idea," said Monica. "I agree."

With that, we all went in to see Mr. Riley: three physicians, three nurses, a social worker and a medical student.

1988

"Who's this?" I asked on rounds one morning, stopping in front of room 4.

"This is Mr. Graham Riley. He's a 37-year-old white male who came in last night with severe pneumonia. Dr. Kotler [the head of Infectious Diseases] wanted him in MICU until his pneumonia is diagnosed and treatment is started. They think he has AIDS."

"I know him," I said. "He was here about nine months ago, also with severe pneumonia. Let me see his old chart."

I picked up his 1987 hospital chart and thumbed through it for a minute. "Here, here's my notes from last year. He was in MICU at that time for bacterial pneumonia. That's when we diagnosed AIDS-Related Complex. He got better and left MICU. Let's see...he was in the hospital a total of three weeks. What happened after he went home? Did he ever get AIDS counselling?"

"Yes," replied Anita, the intern on his case. "Dr. Kotler has been following him in the clinic. He's also received drug-abuse counselling but still admits to using cocaine. Anyway, he was stable until about a week ago when he developed fever and night sweats. He thought it was the flu. He felt so bad last night that he came to the emergency room. His chest x-ray shows diffuse pneumonia. Also, he is very hypoxic, PO-two only fifty-three on room air. They called Dr. Kotler from the Emergency Department and he asked to have him put in MICU."

I looked through the sliding glass doors to see the patient I remembered from last year. He appeared to be about 20 pounds lighter, and every bit as ill as before. It was hard for me to imagine Mr. Riley in a healthy state. This time, I knew, he must have AIDS.

"Did his ARC ever go away?"

"Apparently so," said Anita. "Dr. Kotler says his chest x-ray and lymphadenopathy cleared completely. Mr. Riley was doing well as of last month, when last seen in the clinic. They were monitoring him mainly because of the positive HIV antibody. Dr. Kotler felt it was just a matter of time before he developed AIDS."

"What's the plan?" I asked.

"Dr. Kotler's going to call you this morning, to ask you to bronchoscope him. We've kept him NPO [nothing by mouth] since midnight."

"OK," I said. "Before we go in to see him, let's go look at his chest x-rays."

We walked across the hall to the x-ray reading room. I pulled out his films and put them on the view box.

"Well," I said, "there's little doubt about what's happening here. Compared with the film from 1987, there is a big difference. The 1987 film shows a dense patch of pneumonia in the bottom of his left lung. Now the x-ray shows this diffuse, homogenous pneumonia throughout *both* lungs. Looks like the classic x-ray picture of *pneumocystis carinii* pneumonia."

"I agree." The authoritative voice was that of Dr. Bernie Kotler, head of Memorial's Infectious Disease service. He had just walked into the reading room.   "He needs to be bronchoscoped for confirmation. I'll start him on Bactrim [a drug for PCP] as soon as you finish the bronchoscopy."

"Thanks," I said, with just a hint of sarcasm.

"You're welcome," he replied.

Fiberoptic bronchoscopy involves inserting a thin, flexible tube (the bronchoscope) through the patient's mouth or nose and into the lungs (the bronchi).   A narrow channel through the center of the scope allows suctioning of secretions and removal of tiny biopsies of lung tissue.   In Mr. Riley's case we would be suctioning secretions from the bottom of his lungs for examination under the microscope; the tiny, round *pneumocystis carinii* organisms are visible with special staining.

Bronchoscopy is routine in all acute care hospitals, and is especially useful for diagnosing pneumonia caused by opportunistic-type organisms.   The bronchoscope has a brilliant light on one end; through the other end the examiner can see the inside of the airways and direct the scope almost anywhere in the patient's lungs.

Sooner or later most AIDS patients undergo fiberoptic bronchoscopy, mainly because most AIDS patients develop unusual pneumonia that requires accurate diagnosis. With proper precautions there is virtually no risk of a health worker contracting AIDS during bronchoscopy. We have performed the procedure dozens of times on AIDS patients. Still, AIDS is not the bronchoscopist's favorite diagnosis. No physician wants to become a case report.

*   *   *

We returned to MICU to see Mr. Riley.

"Hi. I'm Dr. Martin. I don't know if you remember me. I took care of you last year when you were here with pneumonia."

He nodded.

"We've discussed your case and it seems that you have another severe pneumonia now. This one is not so easy to diagnose as last year's. We're going to have to do a procedure called bronchoscopy, which involves inserting a thin, flexible tube into your lungs and washing out the area with some saline."

"I know," he said somberly, "they explained it to me last night."

Mr. Riley's physical examination revealed only that he was febrile and chronically ill. His respiratory rate was twice the normal 16 breaths a minute, and he could not tolerate removal of his oxygen mask for more than a few seconds. His lungs were actually clear when listened to with a stethoscope. The exam revealed only that he was very ill and debilitated but gave no clue as to the cause. It was the chest x-ray and positive HIV antibody that made PCP the presumptive diagnosis. Bronchoscopy would confirm that diagnosis or perhaps make another one.

"Let me tell you a little more about the procedure," I said, and continued with the explanation. We obtained his written permission, and a half hour later had the bronchoscope in his lungs. The procedure lasted only ten minutes, enough time to examine both lungs and obtain secretions for microscopic exam.

We had our answer an hour later. Under the microscope was an abundance of *pneumocystis carinii* organisms.

1989

One day during MICU rounds my beeper went off.

"Abe? This is Bernie. Graham Riley is in the ED. He's got grand mal seizures. I suspect he's developed a CNS [central nervous system] infection. I'm sending him for a CAT scan. Do you have a bed in MICU?"

"Sure, Bernie. What do you think he has?"

"I don't know. Could be toxoplasmosis. I'll come to MICU as soon as he's gets there, right after his CAT scan."

"He's not DNR [Do Not Resuscitate], is he?"

"No, not yet," said Bernie. "I've got to talk to his family about that."

Bernie Kotler had followed Mr. Riley for almost two years, from the time we first diagnosed ARC. Mr. Riley had recovered nicely from *pneumocystis carinii* pneumonia in 1988. He had been in the hospital twice since then for other infections, although not in MICU. For the past two months he had received once-a-week pentamidine inhalation treatments to help prevent recurrence of

PCP. Unfortunately pentamidine doesn't prevent numerous other opportunistic infections, several of which can involve the brain. His new onset of seizures now suggested a brain infection.

About an hour after Bernie's phone call Mr. Riley was wheeled into MICU, accompanied by Jill, one of our interns. He was still somnolent from a post-seizure state but was breathing on his own; he was not intubated.

"Well, Jill, what did the CAT scan show?"

"They think its toxoplasmosis," she said.

"How do they know?"

"From the pattern on CAT scan. Dr. Kotler was down there discussing it with the radiologists. He'll be up in a few minutes."

I decided to go see for myself. While they were putting Mr. Riley in a bed I went to the basement and met the radiologist in charge of CAT scanning. He showed me the films.

"These white areas are all abnormal," he said, pointing to several dime-sized spots in Mr. Riley's brain.

"How do you know it's toxoplasmosis?"

"Well, I don't for sure. But given the fact that he has AIDS, it's number one on the list. Theoretically it could be some other infection or even metastatic cancer, but the size and density of these lesions are most compatible with infection."

Toxoplasmosis is infection caused by the protozoan *toxoplasma gondii* which, like *pneumocystis carinii*, is an opportunistic organism too small to see except with the microscope. *Toxoplasma gondii* doesn't infect people with healthy immune systems, so that diagnosis seemed reasonable in view of the CAT scan. And if the cause wasn't toxoplasmosis surely it was some other infection, just as bad. Things didn't look good for Mr. Riley.

"Thanks," I said, and returned to MICU. I met Dr. Kotler at Mr. Riley's bedside.

"You saw the CT scan?" he asked.

"Yes. You think its toxo, right?"

"Well, we have to treat for that."

"Does he need a brain biopsy?"

"No, I don't think so. I've ordered a toxo titer in his blood. That might give a diagnosis. Let's do a spinal tap and send the

CSF [cerebrospinal fluid] for cytology and toxo titers. After that, start him on twenty-five milligrams of pyrimethamine and eight grams of sulfadiazine a day. Also, continue the pentamidine inhalations. If you have the room I'd like him to stay in MICU."

"No problem," I said. "I assume we're to institute any necessary life support, since he's not DNR?"

"For now, that's right. I've discussed this with Mr. Riley already. He wants everything done, but doesn't want to be kept alive on machines if that's the way it ends up. I've got to talk to his family also."

Over the next few days we treated Mr. Riley with drugs for presumed toxoplasmosis of the brain, plus anti-seizure medications and the inhaled pentamidine. On day three he had another grand mal seizure. We stopped the seizure with intravenous Valium, but a few minutes later it recurred: a violent shaking of his entire body. Since he was already on maximal anti-seizure medication there was only one thing left to try — general anesthesia.

Our neurologist on the case recommended intravenous sodium pentothal, a short-acting barbiturate that stops seizures by inducing a deep coma. Since the drug also suppresses breathing the patient must be intubated and receive artificial ventilation. Mr. Riley was intubated and begun on sodium pentothal. Within minutes of beginning the pentothal infusion his seizures stopped.

A repeat brain CAT scan showed some increase in size of the toxoplasmosis lesions. A brain biopsy was considered but ruled out when the blood and spinal fluid titers confirmed infection with *toxoplasma gondii*. Since Mr. Riley did not show any response to standard therapy the dose of each drug was doubled.

On day six Mr. Riley developed pneumonia from *pseudomonas aeruginosa*, a virulent bacteria that infects many chronically ill, hospitalized patients. *Pseudomonas* infection is often very difficult to treat under the best of circumstances and Mr. Riley's AIDS did not make it any easier. We began two additional antibiotics for the pneumonia.

By the end of day seven he was receiving five antibiotics plus intravenous sodium pentothal. Unfortunately his blood gases showed progressive respiratory deterioration from the *pseudomonas* pneumonia.   He required complete ventilatory support and 100% inspired oxygen to maintain a barely adequate blood oxygen level.

The sodium pentothal was temporarily stopped so his EEG could be repeated. As the drug effect wore off the EEG showed a renewal of seizure activity. Pentothal was re-started and he again entered a state of deep coma.

Each day's rounds focused less and less on Mr. Riley's medical therapy and more and more on the ethical issues. By day eight the discussion was almost all ethical.   Three nurses, four physicians (including myself), a medical student, respiratory therapist and social worker were on rounds that day.

"When are we going to stop?" asked Rita, one of the more seasoned ICU nurses. She quickly added, "I mean, isn't it true that AIDS patients in respiratory failure never recover?"

"Well," I said, "the statistics show that the mortality of AIDS patients in an ICU, when at the stage of needing continuous artificial ventilation, is anywhere from eight-five to one hundred percent.   Given Mr. Riley's *pseudomonas* pneumonia, toxo-plasmosis of the brain, and severe respiratory failure, I would say he's closer to one hundred percent."

"Didn't he ask that ventilator support not be continued if it wasn't helping?" asked Rita.

"Yes, that's true," I said. "How many would vote to stop the machine?" Everyone's attention became riveted. My question caught them a little off guard and no one responded.

"I want everyone to respond," I insisted. "There is no right or wrong here. The truth is, the chance for Mr. Riley to recover is close to nil. He did ask Dr. Kotler, before he was admitted to MICU, not to be kept alive on a machine. He's thirty-eight. He has AIDS. Who would stop the machine at this point?"

"Dr. Martin," said Rita, "it doesn't have to be all or nothing, does it? I don't think we can just turn off the ventilator. Can we vote on whether or not to stop the antibiotics and make him DNR, so that we don't add anything else?"

"Yes," I said, "that's more reasonable. Let's vote on whether we should just stop all the heroics and the antibiotics, and keep him on the ventilator. This is just a vote for consensus. We're not going to make a decision right now. OK, who is in favor of cutting back?"

Five hands went up: Rita's, another nurse's, the medical student's, the social worker's, and an intern's, although not the intern caring for Mr. Riley.

"OK. Jan, why don't *you* want to cut back on his care?" Jan was one of our newer, and younger, ICU nurses.

"I don't know," she said. "He's so young. I mean, we do everything for ninety-year-old nursing home patients. It just doesn't seem right to stop treating Mr. Riley."

"OK. Bill, what about you?" Bill was the intern caring for Mr. Riley.

"I don't know either," he said, "I guess I just don't have enough experience to vote one way or the other. This is only my second AIDS patient."

Now Rita spoke up. "What about you Dr. Martin? You have to vote, too."

"Fair enough," I said. "Well, as I said there's no right or wrong. I think you could go either way and not be criticized. My own opinion is that Mr. Riley doesn't have a chance, and that we're wasting valuable resources. However I am personally reluctant to make a decision, for two reasons. First, I don't know his family all that well, at least not as well as Dr. Kotler. Second, I am not an expert on AIDS. Dr. Kotler is. If there is anything experimental in the works, he would know. So the kind of question I've asked will ultimately have to be answered by him. However I do think we should get some guidance on this issue within the next twenty four hours."

On that point everyone agreed.

Followup

Dr. Kotler did decide. After extensive discussion with Mr. Riley's family the decision was made to withdraw antibiotics, since they were not working. The sodium pentothal and ventilator were continued and Mr. Riley was made DNR. Nine days after admission to MICU we transferred him to a regular ward bed. He died on day twelve, from overwhelming infection and shock.

An autopsy revealed extensive toxoplasmosis and destruction of brain tissue, plus severe pneumonia in both lungs.

Mr. Riley was one of 7,450 Americans who succumbed to AIDS in 1989. (For more on AIDS and the AIDS epidemic, see "A Strange Pneumonia," page 39.)

19. As High as a Giraffe's

The top line on Harold Boykin's emergency room ledger was cryptic: "31-yo bm w/ cc severe ha and blurry vis p. wk. Hx from wife."*

> *   Thirty-one-year-old black male with a chief complaint of headache and blurry vision over the past week. History obtained from patient's wife.

The first step in ER triage is to obtain a chief complaint and take vital signs: pulse, respiratory rate, blood pressure. Adele, the ER triage nurse, checked Mr. Boykin's pulse at a regular 80 beats per minute, respirations at 18 per minute. Both were normal. To take his blood pressure she wrapped a cloth cuff around his upper arm and placed her stethoscope bell just below the secured cuff. She placed the other end of the stethoscope in her ears and pumped up the cuff to register 200 mm Hg* on the pressure scale.

> *   Millimeters of mercury, the units for blood pressure. Hg is the chemical symbol for mercury.

This procedure is routine for taking blood pressure. At 200 mm Hg the arm artery is occluded and no blood can get through. With slow deflation of the blood pressure cuff you can hear, via stethoscope, the gentle knocking sound of blood rushing through the partially opened artery. At *that* point the cuff pressure equals the patient's higher or *systolic* blood pressure, normally between 120 and 140 mm Hg. With further cuff deflation blood flows freely through the fully-opened artery and the sounds become inaudible; *that* point represents the patient's lower or *diastolic* blood pressure, normally around 70 to 80 mm Hg.

At 200 mm Hg there should have been silence, but Adele heard the gentle 'knock-knock-knock' of blood rushing through. This meant Mr. Boykin's systolic blood pressure was *higher* than 200. How much higher?

"Let me try again," she said, and deflated the cuff to restore the circulation. Then she pumped the cuff up to 225 mm Hg. Again she heard: 'Knock-knock-knock.'

Adele deflated and then re-inflated the cuff for a third try, this time to 250 mm Hg. 'Knock-knock-knock.' Such an incredibly high pressure! Somewhat in disbelief, Adele looked at Mr. Boykin: "Sir, are you OK?"

Tall, strongly built, with jet black hair and thin mustache, rugged, intelligent face, Harold Boykin did not answer. He stared past the triage nurse, awake, eyes open and showing no distress but obviously unaware of her question. Mrs. Boykin, who had been standing nearby, saw the surprise look in Adele's face.

"Nurse," she asked. "What's wrong? What's wrong with my husband's blood pressure?"

Adele did not answer right away. Instead she reached for the intercom. "Dr. Randall, come to triage please. Dr. Randall, triage, *please!*"

*   *   *

The blood pressure of a giraffe is the highest of all animals, reaching about 300 mm Hg in its systolic, or upper phase, and 200 mm Hg in its diastolic, or lower phase.

Normal *human* blood pressure rises with age: around 120/70 for young adults, up to about 140/90 for those over 65. A blood pressure consistently above 140/90 signifies hypertension in most people. How *much* above 140/90 is used to classify the hypertension as mild, moderate or severe, and to determine treatment.

The giraffe's blood pressure is higher than a human's because the giraffe heart has to pump blood up a neck seven feet long to reach the brain. The human brain, being only about 12 inches above the heart, can be quite nicely served by a much lower pressure.

All blood pressure measurements are recorded relative to mercury, a dense element thirteen times as heavy as water. If your blood pressure is "120 over 70" the pressure in your arteries will support an enclosed column of *mercury* 120 mm Hg high in the systolic phase, and 70 mm Hg high in the diastolic phase.

These values can also be related to water, which is much closer to blood's density than is mercury.

To summarize:

GIRAFFE
- Average distance between adult brain and heart = 7 feet.
- Normal blood pressure = 300/200 mm Hg; this pressure will support a column of *water* 3900 millimeters high (12.8 feet) in the systolic phase and 2600 millimeters high (8.5 feet) in the diastolic phase.

HUMAN
- Average distance between adult head and heart = 12 inches.
- Normal blood pressure = 120/70 mm Hg; this pressure will support a column of *water* 1560 millimeters high (5.1 feet) in the systolic phase and 910 millimeters high (3 feet) in the diastolic phase.

Give the giraffe a human's blood pressure and the animal will die in a state of shock, unable to pump blood to its brain. Give a man a giraffe's blood pressure and he will, if death does not come quickly, at least sustain widespread organ damage.

*   *   *

So-called malignant hypertension — blood pressure high enough to cause damage early in life — has a much higher prevalence in blacks than in other racial groups. The Boykin family has been particularly hard hit. Harold's father died of hypertension-related heart disease at age 58. An older brother is under treatment for the same problem. A sister was hospitalized for severe hypertension (eclampsia) during two pregnancies.

Harold became aware of hypertension at 21, his last year of Army service, when a Medic told him his pressure was high and to "take some pills." He finished his Army duty and was honorably discharged. For the next five years he attended a Veterans' Hospital medical clinic, for blood pressure checks and medication. Control of his pressure was erratic, there were frequent adjustments of medication, yet all the while he felt well. The last drug prescribed affected his libido and was his 'last straw:' too many medications, intolerable side effects, and all for a disease that didn't make him feel bad. Disillusioned, Harold quit attending the clinic and stopped all therapy.

Twice after leaving the veterans' clinic Harold showed up in Memorial's emergency room for flu-related symptoms. On each visit his blood pressure was taken and found elevated and he was advised to attend our hypertension clinic or return to the VA. Twice he ignored the advice.

Then, at age 31, some six years after his last regular therapy for hypertension, Harold developed a severe headache. He made no connection between the headache and high blood pressure, especially since he found some relief with aspirin.

A few days later he complained to his wife of blurry vision *and* persistent headache. Still no connection. Mrs. Boykin actually called the hospital's eye clinic for an appointment, thinking her husband might need glasses. The next day his headache became intolerable and she drove him to Memorial's emergency room.

*   *   *

His blood pressure in the ER was finally measured at 280/180 mm Hg, one of the highest recorded in our hospital. Under Dr. Randall's direction the ER nurses did an electrocardiogram, drew blood and began treatment with under-the-tongue nifedipine, a drug that induces an immediate lowering of blood pressure.

Fifteen minutes after receiving nifedipine Harold's blood pressure was slightly lower, 260/160 mm Hg. In another fifteen minutes it was 250/150. At that point he was transferred to MICU.

On arrival to MICU he appeared in good physical shape, albeit confused. He made no eye contact and did not talk or respond to questions, suggesting swelling of the brain, a potentially fatal condition known medically as *hypertensive encephalopathy*.

We found other stigmata of severe, sustained hypertension: tiny hemorrhages in the back of his eyes (the retina); a large, bounding heart; and protein in his urine. Neurologic exam did not reveal any evidence for stroke or brain hemorrhage (a brain CAT scan was ordered to be sure). Blood drawn in the ER showed diminished kidney function and his electrocardiogram helped confirm an enlarged, hypertrophied heart muscle (cardiomegaly). The damage sustained by his eyes, heart, kidneys, and brain reflected an enormous arterial pounding: the blood pressure of a giraffe in the body of a man.

We started an infusion of *sodium nitroprusside*, the most potent anti-hypertensive agent available. Nitroprusside directly dilates the arterial blood vessels and almost never fails to lower blood pressure.

Because it is so potent nitroprusside is a tricky drug to use. If it lowers blood pressure too much the patient can go into shock from *hypo*tension. If nitroprusside doesn't lower blood pressure enough the patient will remain at high risk for stroke, heart attack, or kidney failure. The goal of nitroprusside therapy is not a normal blood pressure but one that is 'safely elevated,' something on the order of 160/100 mm Hg. The drug's manufacturer cautions:

[Nitroprusside] should be used be used only when the necessary facilities and equipment for continuous monitoring of blood pressure are available.

"Necessary facilities" means an intensive care unit and round-the-clock nursing care. "Equipment for continuous monitoring" usually requires cannulating the patient's radial (or other) artery with a thin catheter. The catheter is connected via plastic tubing to an electronic monitor so arterial pressure can be continuously recorded and digitally displayed at the patient's bedside.

We began infusing two micrograms of nitroprusside per kilogram body weight each minute (notated in the chart as '2 ugm/kg/min'). Within an hour Mr. Boykin's pressure fell to 240/130 mm Hg; within another two hours, 230/122 mm Hg. Still high, but safer.

Intravenous nitroprusside is impractical for long periods and is also potentially dangerous. A metabolite of the drug, thiocyanate, is a cyanide-like compound that can starve the body of oxygen. Cases have been reported of cyanide toxicity from prolonged nitroprusside infusion. We planned only a short course.

The next day Mr. Boykin was awake but still not communicating. On a nitroprusside dose of 3.5 ugm/kgm/minute his blood pressure was down to 200/110 mm Hg. We started him on oral anti-hypertensive drugs and began weaning off the nitroprusside.

*　　*　　*

Most of the 20 million hypertensives in the country never require hospitalization for high blood pressure, let alone intensive care. At Memorial 2-3% of our MICU admissions come in for this problem. Patients needing intensive care for severe hypertension are usually 'new' hypertensives (previously undiagnosed and often with occult kidney disease), or 'known' hypertensives who have been non-compliant with prescribed medication.

If a patient has medication, is compliant in taking it, and receives good followup in the clinic or office, blood pressure can usually be controlled. In fact some patients improve just with a change in life style: weight loss, no smoking, low salt intake, and exercise.

As to drugs, there are many, many choices, from the tried-and-true to the new-and-exotic. Paradoxically, an explosion in the number of medications in recent years has made treatment both easier and more complicated. Easier, because therapy can now be tailored to the individual patient; more complicated, because the sheer number of drugs makes it difficult for doctors to keep up with their nuances and side effects.

For example, captopril, a popular anti-hypertensive drug, is a member of the relatively new ACE-('angiotensin-converting-enzyme') inhibitor group of drugs. Doctors commonly prescribe captopril in place of an older drug type, such as a diuretic, whose side effects may be better appreciated. One recently-recognized side effect of ACE inhibitors is a persistent cough. The cough occurs in a small percentage of patients taking ACE inhibitors, but affects a large number of people because the drugs are widely used. Treatment is to stop the drug and try something else, but first the cough must be appreciated as a drug side effect.

On the next page is a list of oral anti-hypertensive drugs (by no means complete) according to drug type. Under each type the generic drug name is given, followed by brand name(s) in parentheses.

1. DIURETICS
   Furosemide (Lasix)
   Hydrochlorothiazide (Esidrix; HydroDIURIL)
   Chlorothiazide (Diuril)
   Metolazone (Zaroxolyn)

2. CALCIUM CHANNEL BLOCKERS
   Nifedipine (Procardia)
   Verapamil (Calan; Isoptin)
   Diltiazem (Cardizem)
   Nicardipine (Cardene)

3. BETA BLOCKERS
   Atenolol (Tenormin)
   Propranolol (Inderal)
   Timolol (Blocadren)
   Metoprolol (Lopressor)
   Betaxolol (Kerlone)

4. ACE INHIBITORS
   Captopril (Capoten)
   Enalapril (Vasotec)
   Lisinopril (Zestril)

5. MISCELLANEOUS:
   Prazosin (Minipress)
   Clonidine (Catapres)
   Methyldopa (Aldomet)
   Hydralazine (Apresoline)

A *single* drug is usually prescribed for mild to moderate elevations of blood pressure. *Two or more drugs* are used for severe cases or when hypertension doesn't respond to a single agent. The actual dose of any drug depends on the patient's tolerance and response. Given the type and number of available drugs, plus the range of dosages, hundreds of outpatient regimens can be formulated.

*   *   *

By the middle of Mr. Boykin's second day in MICU we were able to stop nitroprusside infusion and continue therapy with just two oral medications, Catapres and Lasix. His brain CAT scan showed no bleeding or stroke so we expected decent recovery from the encephalopathy.

By day three his blood pressure was 170/105 and the encephalopathy had cleared. For the first time in four days Harold Boykin was alert *and* oriented. I had my first discussion with him that afternoon.

"How do you feel?" I asked.

"Much better," he said, without affect. In fact I was struck by his lack of emotion on this point, certainly none of the glad-to-be-alive aura we see in some patients. Either he was sullen by nature or perhaps still somewhat depressed by the effects of encephalopathy.

"Mr. Boykin, do you know what happened?"

"I guess my blood pressure was high. That's what the nurses tell me."

"How long have you known about this blood pressure problem?"

"They found it when I was in the Army. That was about ten years ago.

"Do you know how serious it is?" To that question he looked at me for a few seconds, as if to say, 'What do you think, I'm some kind of jerk?' and I felt a little self conscious asking these leading questions.

"I guess pretty serious. I wouldn't have all these tubes in me if it wasn't." (He still had an arterial line and a venous infusion catheter).

He didn't object to my questions so I decided to press ahead. "Mr. Boykin, you almost died from it. As it is, your heart is enlarged and your kidneys show damage from the blood pressure."

His attitude remained rather sullen. He had evidently heard such threats before. Now I was telling him *faits accompli*; these things had happened. The doctors hadn't been kidding all these years.

"Will they get better?" he asked, with about as little emotion as if one asked 'Where is the men's room?'

"We don't know yet. Your pressure's only been down a short time now. We have to wait and see if any of the damage is reversible. That might take several weeks. You won't stay here, of course. You'll have to start coming to the clinic regularly. Why did you stop taking your medication?"

"I didn't have any to take."

"I mean several years ago, when you were being treated."

"I don't know. That was a long time ago. I remember the medicine made me sick. I actually felt better without it."

"Your wife told me you also smoke."

"Yes, I do."

"How much?"

"About a pack a day."

"How long?"

"Since I was a teenager, I guess."

I paused for a few seconds. Staring him in the eyes, I said: "I don't know if anyone's ever told you before, but you're a walking time bomb."

"What do you mean?"

"Well, what usually kills hypertensive patients like you is a heart attack or stroke. You came very close to having a stroke the day you came in, do you know that?"

"Now that you tell me I do."

* * *

I don't enjoy preaching to patients. So many of them are sick because they drink or smoke too much, or use illicit drugs, or don't take their prescribed medications. My Boykin's problems, tobacco addiction and hypertension, are in theory preventable or treatable, like alcoholism and cocaine abuse. Stop drinking, stop smoking, stop abusing drugs. It all sounds so simple *in theory*. The reality is far different.

Intensive care specialists take pride in bringing a diabetic out of coma or rescuing a hypertensive from the brink of death or weaning a patient away from artificial ventilation. The pride may be justified but we should ask on each occasion: would the coma, encephalopathy or respiratory failure have occurred in the first place if there was better outpatient care, more patient education, effective drug rehab programs?

It is one thing to treat an acute, life-threatening illness and another to prevent the problem. The latter is the real challenge. Compared to good outpatient care for patients like Harold Boykin, that is, compared to effective *preventive medicine*, intensive care is easy.

Followup

On the fourth day in MICU Mr. Boykin's blood pressure was down to 160/95 and we transferred him to the regular ward. He stayed another week in the hospital.

Unfortunately his kidneys were irreversibly impaired, almost to the point of requiring kidney dialysis. A hypertension specialist took over his outpatient management and prescribed a regimen to help preserve remaining kidney function. The regimen included a low-salt diet and three anti-hypertensive drugs: Catapres, Lasix, and Minipress.

Perhaps frightened by events, Mr. Boykin has become very compliant. He now regularly attends the hypertension clinic and takes his medication. He knows that blood pressure pills are the only thing keeping him from a suffering a stroke, heart attack, or life-long kidney dialysis.

20. Ascending Weakness

Thirty-five-year-old Naomi Benedict was sitting in a chair at home, recovering from the flu, when she felt a sudden tingling in both legs. She stood up to stretch, lost her balance and promptly fell to the floor.

The maid ran in from the kitchen. What was wrong? Mrs. Benedict said the only problem was that her legs felt weak and tingly, as if their circulation was cut off. Otherwise she felt fine. The maid helped her stand up, then climb the stairs to the bedroom and get into bed.

It was two in the afternoon on Tuesday, March 7. Mr. Benedict, an attorney, was at work and their two young children were in school. At three o'clock she was to attend the city's Arts Council meeting, her first time out in a week. Instead of getting dressed she lay in bed, unsure what to do.

She called her husband. Julian Benedict thought her leg weakness was probably from the flu and sitting too long in one position. He suggested she call Dr. Cooper and not try to make the meeting.

Dr. Cooper, one of the town's leading internists, knew the Benedicts well as both their physician and friend. He advised her to stay in bed; if not substantially better in the morning, after a good night's sleep, she should come to his office.

The next morning I was in MICU making rounds, when Dr. Cooper phoned.

"Larry, I've got Naomi Benedict in my office. You know who she is, don't you?"

"Sure," I said, "her husband is Julian Benedict, right? I've seen their picture in the magazines." I did not know them personally but I knew *of* them. At the time he was a rising young lawyer, famous after his defense of a business tycoon charged with murder. When his client won acquittal Julian Benedict's name was all over the papers. At age 39 he was a legal star.

I was aware of Naomi as a young socialite and heiress to a family fortune made in the steel industry. Like many young and wealthy women she was active in prominent charities, one of which made donations to Memorial Hospital. She and her husband were also well known, at least locally, because of their home. 'La Maison Magnifique', so dubbed by an overly enthusiastic editor, was featured in the city magazine four months earlier. The Benedicts had spent a fortune redecorating an old French chateau-style mansion into something that, even by European standards, was stunning (at least from the pictures; I have never been inside). Naomi's college degree was in art history and she had orchestrated the entire project.

"Well, I've been treating her for a viral gastro-enteritis the past week," Dr. Cooper continued. "She had the flu with some diarrhea and was getting better, at least until yesterday. She had a little leg weakness yesterday and this morning can hardly walk. I'm not sure, but it might be progressive. She also has some diminished breath sounds. I did a vital capacity [a measure of lung function] in the office and it's down to about 70% of predicted. Larry, I'm worried about her. I'd like to put her in MICU if you have a bed."

Dr. Cooper is known for good medical judgment so if he worries about a patient I do too. "Of course," I said. "We'll get a bed ready for her. When do you think she'll be here?"

"Well, Julian's with her and he'll bring her down to the hospital. With her difficulty walking, it'll take them about half an hour."

"OK. We'll be ready."

A few minutes later Harold McAllister, Memorial's Director of Neurology, stopped by. Just past 40, tall and aristocratic in bearing, Harold is a neurologist's neurologist, which is to say he regularly consults on the rich and famous. Even in the era of CAT and magnetic resonance scanners, neurologic diagnosis is an art based on thorough history and detailed physical examination. Dr. McAllister is an artist.

"Hello Harold, what's up? Who are you here to see?"

"No one just yet. I understand Naomi Benedict is being admitted soon."

"Yes, that's right. Did Dr. Cooper call you also?"

"He left a message with my secretary to see her right away.

When do you expect her?"

"Within the hour. I just talked to Cooper a few minutes ago."

"OK. Would you please page me as soon as she arrives?"

"Sure."

A few minutes later the Chief of the Department of Medicine walked in. He pulled me aside from rounds, to speak privately.

"Larry, Naomi Benedict is coming to MICU. She apparently has. . ."

"I know," I interrupted, somewhat surprised by this unexpected visit from my boss. "I spoke with Dr. Cooper a while ago and Harold McAllister was just here also."

"Well, I just came to tell you about Julian, her husband. I don't think you know him. He's on the hospital's board of trustees. (Dr. Cooper hadn't mentioned this.) He's one of the nicest guys you'll ever meet, a tiger in court but outside the courtroom he's a real gentleman. Naomi works on the hospital's auxiliary. I can't tell you how much money she's helped raise for Memorial. I know them both. Don't be intimidated by their wealth or position. They are down-to-earth people. She, especially, is a doll. I sure hope she's OK. Maybe Cooper is just being over cautious. Anyway, call me if you need assistance of any kind. We want to do everything necessary to help her."

I wanted to reply that "everything necessary" is what we do for all our patients, but instead just thanked the Chief for his well-intentioned advice. Some degree of anxiety is natural when VIPs (or their relatives) become patients. Socially prominent people, including politicians, business leaders, and movie stars, always expect (and usually receive) special treatment. The difference is in nuances of service, not in basic medical care. In fact, doctors sometimes have to be careful not to let 'VIP care' affect sound medical practice. A desire not to intrude, not to bother, can sometimes inhibit doctors from doing an important test or procedure, although this is less likely to happen in MICU. I learned long ago that all patients, whether dope addict or corporation president, or the rich wife of a hot shot trial lawyer, want (and deserve) the same thing: good medical care delivered in a friendly and compassionate manner.

A few minutes later the swinging doors to MICU opened and

an attendant ushered in Mrs. Benedict in a wheel chair. Julian Benedict walked beside her. From TV and magazine photos I recognized them right away, although Julian appeared shorter than I had imagined. A three piece business suit covered his stocky, muscular frame. Clean shaven, tie perfectly knotted, he appeared ready to go to court. Naomi, also smartly dressed in street clothes, carried a purse on her lap.

Unlike most patients admitted to MICU she was fully alert and in no distress. My first thought was that perhaps she didn't need to be in MICU, that she might be more comfortable in a private room in one of the hospital towers. My second thought was that the towers are not equipped to closely monitor patients, and if Dr. Cooper wanted close observation she probably should be in MICU.

The MICU nurses went right to work. Since the Benedicts had bypassed normal admission procedures they sent Mr. Benedict to the admitting office, to provide insurance information and sign some papers. Then they took Mrs. Benedict into room 2 and exchanged her street clothes for a hospital gown. After a few minutes Emily, one of the RN's, came out to get a bed scale. She gave me a knowing smile.

"Why the look?" I asked.

"Anne Klein skirt and blouse? Gucci shoes and purse? Can you believe it?"

I acted dumb. "Is that fancy?"

A rhetorical question, at least for Emily. She changed her expression to show that I was quite out of touch, and returned to Mrs. Benedict's room.

Since Mrs. Benedict could not stand up the nurses measured her height lying supine (five feet five inches). Next, they recorded temperature (normal), blood pressure (125/72), heart rate (105 beats per minute), respiratory rate (18 breaths a minute — normal), and skin turgor (normal); hoisted her on a stretcher over the bed to obtain her weight (129 pounds); and attached EKG monitor leads to her chest. From that moment her heart rate and rhythm were continuously displayed on a bedside monitor.

When the nurses finished I put in a page for Dr. McAllister and, accompanied by Janice Dover, one of the MICU interns, went in to see our new patient. Even without the fancy clothes she was so different from our usual intensive care patient (elderly or debilitated or acutely ill). Here in MICU was a very attractive woman: light complexion, brown hair combed straight back, little makeup, with the poise and bearing of a top fashion model. Even in the bare cloth of a hospital gown, without jewelry, she looked elegant, not unlike Jackie Onassis at a similar age.

"Mrs. Benedict, I'm Dr. Martin and this is Dr. Dover. I run the ICU and Dr. Dover is one of our interns. Dr. Cooper called me when you were in his office and told us something of your problem."

She smiled, then spoke with a mixture of embarrassment and concern. "Hello. I feel so foolish being here. Do you really think the intensive care unit is necessary? I don't feel sick."

"Well, Dr. Cooper is worried about your sudden weakness."

"I know. I just can't walk. I feel so helpless. What do you think it is?"

"We don't know yet. He wants us to watch you for a day or so and run some tests. If there is no progression of the weakness you'll go home or to another part of the hospital to recuperate. He's also asked the head of our Neurology division to see you. That's Dr. McAllister. He will be down in a few minutes."

"Can my husband come in for just a minute? I want to tell him not to wait around. It's not necessary."

I checked her vital signs from the nurse's records. They were all normal except for the slightly fast heart rate. "Sure, I'll go see if he's through in the admitting office."

Julian returned to MICU and went in to see his wife. He came out five minutes later and announced he was leaving the hospital for a few hours. Apparently she had insisted that he go to work and come back in the afternoon, when more would be known about her condition. There would be no problem with the kids, since the Benedicts had a full-time housekeeper.

About this time Dr. McAllister returned to MICU. Consultants on new admissions don't usually appear until after the intern has examined the patient, but in this case Dr. McAllister was asked to get involved right away. He apologized for "intruding" so soon, and suggested we interview her together, then let him do the neurologic exam. This approach was reasonable since it would obviate repetition of her medical history.

Dr. McAllister introduced himself and began eliciting her story, the outline of which is related above. Mrs. Benedict had no trouble speaking or recalling events leading up to hospitalization. She impressed us as bright and articulate and, for all the press hype, remarkably free of affectation, an ordinary (if rich) human being who wanted nothing more than to get better and go home. On a personal level I felt sorry for her.

Accustomed to all the druggies, alcoholics, and non-compliant patients we routinely see, as well as those in coma or serious distress, her presence in MICU seemed anomalous. She was not even sick. I couldn't get the idea out of my head: what is she *doing* here? Her weakness could progress, but in the scheme of things why should it? She hadn't done anything 'bad' to justify a serious illness. No drugs, no alcohol, no promiscuity.

But of course these were foolish thoughts. There are many more diseases than those brought on by self-abuse. I reflected on Eric Siegel's *Love Story* and its depressing ending: innocence and happiness dashed by cruel fate. Mrs. Benedict was innocent. She had caught a virus and developed muscle weakness. Now, she could crash just like any other patient with a bad disease.

Another question from Dr. McAllister interrupted my ruminations. "Mrs. Benedict, did you run a fever when you had the flu?"

"I took my temperature only twice. Once, at the beginning of the flu, it was a hundred and one. Two or three days later it was down to one hundred. I haven't taken it since but I think I'm recovered from the flu. At least I feel better."

"Before you developed leg weakness, that is before yesterday, did you have any numbness or tingling of your arms or legs?"

"No. The weakness and tingly feeling came on at the same time."

"Have the numbness and tingling persisted?"

"Yes. My legs have a tingling feeling now, like they're still asleep."

"But you have sensation in your legs? You can feel the bed

sheets?"

"Yes, but my legs feel almost like they're not part of me, like they're still asleep."

"Have you had any trouble breathing?"

"No. Well, wait a minute. Yesterday I did feel a little short of breath after climbing the stairs. And this morning, getting into the car, I guess I was a little winded, but that's all. It's probably because I feel so tired."

"Do you smoke?"

"No, not at all"

"How about your husband?"

"Smoke? No, Julian doesn't smoke either."

"Have you ever had any respiratory problems, pneumonia, asthma, any lung trouble before?"

"No, nothing. This is actually the first time I've been in the hospital since Kevin [their younger child] was born. That was six years ago. In fact, I felt great until last week."

"Do you do any regular exercise?"

"Yes! Doubles tennis. Twice a week."

"When was the last time you played?"

"Two weeks ago. I haven't played since I got the flu."

"There was no fall-off in your game? I mean, the last time you played, did everything seem normal in your game?"

Here she gave a little laugh. "Yes. I mean, we lost, but I felt fine."

"Other than the weakness in your legs, have you noticed weakness anywhere else?"

She opened and closed her fists a few times. "No, I feel fine everywhere else."

"Has your weakness increased since yesterday? Is it harder for you to walk this morning than when you first noticed the weakness?"

"Yes. Yesterday, even after I fell on the floor I could walk a little. This morning my legs were weaker. Julian had to practically carry me into and out of the car. I could not make it by myself. Now I couldn't walk if I had to."

"Have you had any problem with your period? Is it regular?"

"Yes."

"Any history of kidney or heart disease?"

"No, none."

"How about arthritis?"

"No."

"Do you take any medication?"

"No, only what Dr. Cooper prescribed last week."

"What was that?"

"Erythromycin [an antibiotic] and some Donnatal [an anti-spasmodic for the diarrhea]."

"You've taken no other drugs the past few months?"

"Oh, an occasional aspirin. But nothing else."

"Have you eaten anything rotten or that tasted rotten in the past few weeks?"

"No. Nothing. Do you think this could be food poisoning?"

"Probably not.   Botulism — and I *don't* think you have botulism — can sometimes present with progressive weakness."

There were several more questions about possible exposure to insect spray, toxic chemicals, and other people with similar afflictions, but the answers were all negative. In essence her history was straightforward: a healthy and active woman; flu-like illness for about a week; development of abrupt leg weakness; progression over the ensuing 18 hours.

Next came the neurologic exam. Dr. McAllister was a marvel to watch as he tested her sense of smell and taste, eye movements in all directions, strength of muscles from neck to toes, reflexes, and numerous other aspects of nerve function. His exam was meticulous, thorough, and kind. He explained any poke or prod that might cause some discomfort. (He did not concentrate on her heart, lungs, or abdomen, as these organ systems are not part of a neurologic exam; Dr. Dover and myself would return to check these areas.)

Apart from her lower extremities the neurologic exam was "unremarkable." Her legs revealed the problem. Normally we can push our toes down (a motion called 'dorsiflexion') with great strength, as when pushing against a bed board or standing on our tip toes; Mrs. Benedict could not push down at all. While lying flat we can lift our legs into the air and hold them up for at least a few seconds. She could not lift her legs even a fraction of an inch. We can easily take one leg and cross it over the other, from knee to ankle. This, too, she could not do. All she could accomplish with either leg was a slight rolling motion on the bed sheet.

She had sensation in both legs and could feel Dr. McAllister's warm hands and the gentle prick of his safety pin. Also of diagnostic importance was the *absence* of muscle reflexes in her legs. Normally there is a reflex jerking of the leg if the knee is tapped with a rubber hammer. Her legs didn't budge.

After the history and exam, which took about an hour, we thanked her and went to the nurses' station.

"What do you think?" Dr. McAllister asked Dr. Dover.

"Well, she can't dorsiflex [push down] her feet, so there's weakness there. It looks like a primary motor weakness of the lower extremities."

"Exactly," he commented. "And coming on a week after a viral illness, it makes you think of one particular diagnosis."

"Guillain-Barré syndrome?"

"Very good, Dr. Dover! Yes, she has the classic picture of Guillain Barré syndrome. The weakness began in her feet and seems to be progressing upwards. Now her thigh muscles are weak. Frankly, I'm also a little worried about her breathing. Larry, I didn't detect any respiratory muscle weakness but that can happen if this progresses any further. We should check her vital capacity several times a day. Until we see which way she's going I definitely want her to stay here. In the meantime we'll need to do an LP [lumbar puncture] and an EMG [electromyogram] to help secure the diagnosis."

*   *   *

Georges Guillain and Jean A. Barré, two early 20th century French neurologists, were among the first to describe inflammation of the peripheral nerves leading to paralysis. They recognized that the paralysis occurred most commonly after a respiratory infection. Today the eponym 'Guillain-Barré' is widely used for the syndrome of post-infection paralysis.

In GBS myelin sheaths covering the motor nerves are

damaged. An analogy is the rubber sheath around a thin piece of metal wire that, when damaged, prevents the wire from transmitting electricity. In GBS the myelin sheath is damaged and the nerve does not transmit impulses. The specific mechanism is unknown, although it is probably related to antibodies generated by the infectious agent (usually a virus).

GBS usually afflicts men more than women, and can strike at any age. The most benign cases show only minor muscle weakness and then remit altogether. The most severe cases result in total paralysis. If the myelin sheaths regenerate, which happens in the majority of cases, and the patient doesn't die from acute respiratory or cardiac failure, the prognosis for recovery is good. Joseph Heller, the celebrated author of *Catch 22*, developed severe paralysis from GBS and recovered.

GBS classically presents as *ascending paralysis*, meaning it starts in the legs and progresses up the body. Atypically, paralysis can start in the head (with facial and eye muscle weakness, for example) and *descend*, or start in the middle of the body (arm weakness) and travel both ways. The worst fear is paralysis of the respiratory (breathing) muscles. To have some idea what this type of respiratory failure is like do the following. Stop breathing without 'holding your breath.' Instead, keep your mouth and throat open but do not move your chest (rib) cage. Keep your chest perfectly still. When you can no longer do so, notice how much your chest cage moves as you take in the very next breath. If you couldn't move your chest you would asphyxiate (in about four minutes).

The totally paralyzed patient cannot breathe because the chest cage doesn't move; without movement there is no expansion of the lungs. Without lung expansion no fresh air enters the blood. All such patients require artificial ventilation, for as long as the paralysis lasts.

Examination of the spinal canal fluid — the clear liquid that bathes the spinal cord — can help secure the diagnosis of GBS. Spinal fluid is removed for analysis through a hollow needle inserted in the middle of the back at the level of the hips. (Reach around your back to the spine just between your hips. With the tips of your fingers feel the protuberances of the spinal column.

In a spinal tap the needle goes between these two protuberances.)
A few drops of spinal fluid are removed and sent to the lab for
analysis of protein, glucose, and cell count. A spinal tap is
technically not difficult and is often done by housestaff.

*   *   *

"I better do the spinal tap," said Dr. McAllister, "but it doesn't
have to be done right away. Why don't you finish your workup,
then call me. By the way, I met Mr. Benedict on his way out. I'll
talk to him again when he comes back this afternoon."

Dr. Dover and I returned to finish the physical exam. Apart
from the neurologic system everything was normal. We also drew
blood for routine tests and did the vital capacity measurement.
Our exam and tests took about 45 minutes.

Afterwards I paged Dr. McAllister. He returned to MICU and
obtained permission from Mrs. Benedict for the spinal tap. The
major complication, he explained, is 'post-spinal' headache, which
occurs in perhaps 15% of patients.

While she lay on one side he injected a local anesthetic into a
small area of skin over the spinal column. In a few minutes the
area was fully numb. He then inserted an .18 gauge spinal needle
into the space between two vertebral bodies. The needle entered
her spinal canal with a slight 'give.' Success. Out flowed crystal
clear spinal fluid. One...two... three...four cc's. The precious fluid
was collected and the needle withdrawn. Mrs. Benedict reported
no pain from the procedure.

"I'll check the lab results," he said, "and call Dr. Cooper to let
him know how she's doing. In the meantime, please page me
when Mr. Benedict arrives. By the way, were you able to get the
vital capacity?"

"Yes. It's slightly low," I said. "Three point two liters. We
also did an arterial blood gas, which is normal."

In four hours we had accomplished a battery of tests and
exams that would have taken much longer on the general medical
ward. We had also made a tentative diagnosis and plan of action,
and set up a chart of items to follow her course: muscle strength
of upper and lower extremities; vital capacity; respiratory rate;

body temperature; blood pressure; and heart rate.

Those first few hours convinced me she was in the right place. Ascending paralysis can move fast. Doctors and nurses have to be prepared to move faster.

*   *   *

She went rapidly downhill. By four p.m., slightly over 24 hours after the onset of leg weakness and six hours after arriving in MICU, she began losing strength in her arms. More ominous, her respiratory rate increased to 28 breaths per minute and vital capacity fell to 2.1 liters. I met with Dr. McAllister.

"What do you think?" I asked.

"She's progressing, no doubt about it," he said. "I'm going to start plasmapheresis right away."

"Can that reverse such a rapid slide?"

"Sometimes yes, sometimes no. It's best if plasmapheresis is started before the patient ends up on a ventilator. The sooner the better. There was a large-scale study a few years ago on plasmapheresis in GBS. Something like 250 patients [Neurology, August 1985, volume 35, pages 1096-1104]. They found definite improvement in patients who received plasmapheresis. But you have to start it early in the course."

"Aren't you surprised by how fast she's progressing?"

"Yes I am. GBS usually progresses over a few days or weeks, rarely over a few hours. I've seen one other patient progress this fast. And there are some cases like this in the literature. Cooper sure knew what he was doing by putting her in MICU."

Dr. McAllister called the plasmapheresis service. The physician in charge agreed with the plan and arranged for technicians to begin pheresis that same evening.

They didn't get a chance. As Dr. McAllister was hanging up the phone an alarm went off in Mrs. Benedict's room. We ran in. Her pulse was 160 and she was *very short of breath*.

"Dr. Martin!" she gasped.

I was shocked by the change. Neck muscles contracted with each breath and her skin was mottled and blue. Her speech was short, interrupted, gasping.

"What's. . .the matter?. . .What's happening to me?. . .Why can't I. . .breathe?"

Paralysis had ascended so rapidly that her diaphragm, the major breathing muscle that sits between the abdomen and chest, was now totally paralyzed. She was breathing only with 'backup' neck muscles, and those were about to fail.

I spoke quickly to the nurse. "Please hand me the Ambu bag. And call anesthesia. She needs to be intubated right away!" I began manual Ambu ventilation with 100% oxygen through a tight-fitting face mask. This would keep her going until we could get her intubated.

"Just breathe through this mask, Mrs. Benedict. You'll be fine," I reassured her.

Patients who can't breathe because of *lung* disease usually flail their arms and move their chest cage rapidly in and out. Mrs. Benedict did not have lung failure; her lungs, the organs of respiration inside the chest cage, were normal. Her respiratory muscles had failed and she could not expand her chest. There was *no* movement of her chest (except when some air was pushed in by my squeezing the Ambu bag). Without artificial breathing assistance she would die.

The anesthesiologist came right away and intubated her with a foot-long, 1/4-inch-wide plastic tube; one end of the tube stuck out from her mouth and the other end disappeared inside her throat. With the tube in place we had a secure airway and as soon as we connected the tube to the ventilator she 'pinked up.' The ventilator — replete with alarms and constantly monitored by technicians — was now her life support.

A quick physical exam uncovered no permanent damage. Blood pressure, heart rate, skin perfusion were all OK. But what a close call! She almost died and I felt certain *she* knew this.

I checked an arterial blood gas, which was adequate, then called Dr. Cooper and Mr. Benedict. Both men said the same thing: "I'll be right down."

* * *

Julian went in to visit his wife. I also went in the room, mainly to observe the cardiac monitor in case there was an autonomic surge. Despite modest sedation Naomi's mind was completely intact. The distress of being fully aware yet unable to speak or move could lead to tachycardia.

"Naomi, this is Julian. Can you hear me?"

For the moment she lay there, motionless, eyes closed, a beautiful woman with a tube in her throat, surrounded by machines and monitors and wires.

"Julian, give her a gentle nudge," I said.

He touched her shoulder. "Naomi, this is Julian. Can you hear me?"

She opened her eyes and nodded her head, slowly.

"Hi, honey. The kids send their love. I told them you're doing fine. It's five o'clock now. They're home with Gertrude, eating supper."

A tear came to her eyes.

"We miss you, honey. You'll be home soon. The doctors say this paralysis is a short term thing, that it's completely reversible. Do you understand what I'm saying?"

More tears. And in Julian's eyes, too. I wiped Naomi's tears away with a towel. It was an awkward moment and I wanted to leave them alone. Her heart rhythm looked stable on the monitor so I left the room. Julian emerged about ten minutes later, his face freshly washed. Neither of us said a word.

Just then Dr. McAllister appeared. The three of us went into a MICU conference room, a small, square space almost completely filled with a round wood table. I hastily moved books and journals off the table. We sat down and I led off the discussion.

"Obviously her condition has progressed, much faster than anyone expected. Unfortunately one of the worst things has happened, the paralysis has affected her breathing muscles. She is stable but right now can't breathe without the ventilator. We plan to start a treatment called plasmapheresis, to wash out antibodies from her blood."

"What's that?" he said quickly.

Dr. McAllister answered. "As Dr. Martin said, it's a technique that removes plasma and gets rid of antibodies that might be damaging her nerves. We think antibodies against the nerves are responsible for destroying the myelin sheaths or nerve coverings. We wash out the antibodies with a series of plasma exchanges over two weeks, five or six treatments total. It's fairly safe and there are relatively few complications."

"Does she have to receive blood transfusions with this?"

"No, not at all. We infuse albumin to replace the plasma that's removed. There's no risk of AIDS or hepatitis, if that's what you're concerned about."

"And you say two weeks?"

"Yes. That's the standard length of time most patients are treated. We probably won't see much improvement before two weeks either."

Mr. Benedict did not react to this information. Instead he looked at me and asked, "Dr. Martin, you said 'one of the worst' things. What's the worst?"

"Well, people can die from Guillain Barré syndrome. I think you know that. It usually happens not from the paralysis itself, because we can support her breathing indefinitely, but from what we call autonomic dysfunction. The autonomic part of the nervous system controls things like heart rate and blood pressure. We don't understand why, but sometimes people with this condition can have a sudden surge of adrenalin. This can cause severe blood pressure swings and cardiac arrhythmia. If there is no autonomic crisis, and her nerve coverings regenerate as they usually do, she can fully recover. That's what we're aiming for, of course."

Mr. Benedict addressed Dr. McAllister. "I know her breathing is impaired but is there any sign of recovery in the rest of her body?"

"No, but that's not surprising. It's usually progressive paralysis and then recovery, rather than some areas getting better while others get worse. Right now I'd say she's nowhere near the recovery phase. We probably won't see any definite improvement for a week or more, even with plasmapheresis."

"I see," he said. "Well, the kids want to see their Mom. I told them they can't see her now because she has a bad infection and they might catch it. I really don't want them to see her like this, but if she improves can they visit her here?"

"Sure," I said, "but I agree now's not the time. It would be much better when she's more awake and can interact with them. In fact, if there is no dramatic improvement in the next two days I'm going to recommend a tracheostomy. That will allow us to take the endotracheal tube out of her mouth and put it through a small hole in her neck. Then she can eat, smile, and stay on the ventilator as long as necessary."

"She might not be able to eat just yet," interjected Dr. McAllister. "Sometimes this condition can affect the swallowing muscles. I wouldn't be surprised if hers are already involved, the way this thing has progressed."

He was right, of course. I should have thought of swallowing difficulty before saying she could eat with the tracheostomy. "That's true," I corrected. "But I would still recommend a tracheostomy for reasons of comfort."

"Well," replied Mr. Benedict, "let's cross that bridge when we come to it."

Plasmapheresis was started that evening. There was no immediate response (none was expected so soon) and she remained ventilator-dependent. In fact, her paralysis progressed and by the next morning she could not move even her head. Only her eyes moved. We took advantage of this last vestige of motor function to teach her to answer 'yes' (eyes up and down) and 'no' (side to side).

Dr. Dover inserted a thin stomach tube through her nose for tube feedings. Other tubes already inserted included large intravenous lines for the plasmapheresis and a bladder catheter for collecting urine.

There was no change in her condition after 48 hours. I called Mr. Benedict about the need for tracheostomy and he gave permission. The operation was done on Thursday afternoon by a surgeon. She returned from the operating room with the tracheostomy tube in place and her face free of any encumbrance.

By the end of the third day we had results of several tests, all of which confirmed or were consistent with GBS. The spinal fluid protein was slightly elevated. Since the protein content reaches a peak value several days into the illness, Dr. McAllister thought the small rise merely reflected an early measurement. An EEG or electroencephalogram, done the day after she 'crashed', was normal except for some mild sedative effect, again consistent with GBS. The EEG is a test of brain wave activity and not of peripheral nerves impulses like the EMG. Her EMG showed normal muscles but abnormal nerve conduction within the muscles, the type of impairment typically seen in GBS.

* * *

On the evening of the third day, about one hour after her second plasmapheresis, the nurses turned her to change the bed sheets. Almost immediately Mrs. Benedict's heart rate increased from 95 to 160 per minute and blood pressure bottomed out at 65/30. The nurses quickly rolled her back and pushed a button to lower the head of the bed to the Trendelenburg position. (Named after the German surgeon Friedrick Trendelenburg. In this position the body is angled about 30 degrees with the head down, to facilitate blood flow to the brain.)

The MICU resident reacted swiftly to the autonomic crisis. She ordered a "wide open" saline infusion and intravenous verapamil, a drug that can slow a too-rapidly beating heart. These measures worked and in five minutes her blood pressure was up to 110/64 and heart rate down to 112 a minute. I was not in MICU at the time but it didn't matter; I could not have done a better job. (For the next few days the nurses were advised to turn Mrs. Benedict very slowly and with an eye on the monitor).

On Saturday, March 11, Dr. McAllister and I again met with Mr. Benedict. "As you can see she's doing about the same," I said. "Since last night's episode of low blood pressure she's been quite stable. She still needs the ventilator and will probably stay on it for some time."

"We're going to continue the plasmapheresis another week to ten days," added Dr. McAllister. "By then we should see some improvement, although I must tell you I have seen paralysis continue for months before there is significant nerve sheath regeneration."

Julian listened intently, then spoke. This time it was he who

had something to tell us. "A member of my firm did some work
for one of the New York hospitals. He made some inquiries
when I told him about Naomi's condition and obtained the name
of a neurologist there. I hope you two don't mind if this doctor
consults on Naomi."

"Not at all, not at all," said Dr. McAllister, mildly surprised.

"It's certainly OK with me," I added.

"Who is it?" asked Dr. McAllister.

"A fellow named X____."

At this Dr. McAllister raised his eyebrows. "Well, you
certainly picked a winner. He's probably the world's top authority
on GBS. I've heard him speak several times."

"Good. I didn't know you knew him, but I'm glad you have no
objection. I trust you guys implicitly. I wouldn't be on the Board
if I didn't think this is a damn good hospital. I have to do this for
myself. If for some reason Naomi doesn't make it I want to know
I did everything possible."

"I understand perfectly," said Dr. McAllister. "When's he
coming in?"

"Tomorrow. He could only come on Sunday. I'm picking him
up at the airport tomorrow morning."

* * *

That afternoon I went to the library and read most of Dr. X's
recent papers on Guillain Barré syndrome. Although our
specialties were different I didn't want to seem ignorant of his
work. His publications were mostly clinical, dealing with natural
history of the disease, effect of various treatments, and long term
followup of patients. In these areas he was an authority on GBS.

There was no change in Mrs. Benedict's condition all day
Saturday. On Sunday Mr. Benedict and his New York consultant
showed up in MICU about 11 a.m. Dr. X, about 50, was wearing
a casual sport coat without tie, and comfortable loafers. His
personality seem to match: low key, self-assured, friendly. The
only thing he brought with him was a large brief case full of
neurologic testing equipment. I wondered what he was charging
for this out-of-town visit, on what was most likely his day off.

Whatever the fee, it probably didn't matter to Mr. Benedict.

I handed him Mrs. Benedict's hospital chart and x-ray folder. "I'll be in the hospital," I said. "If you have any questions just ask one of the nurses to page me." He thanked me graciously and went to read her file.

Dr. X spent much of Sunday afternoon in MICU, examining Mrs. Benedict and reviewing the hospital record, then talking with me, Dr. McAllister and Mr. Benedict. In essence he agreed with our evaluation and plans. As far as he was concerned she had a confirmed case of Guillain Barré syndrome.

The consultant recognized his main job was to reassure Mr. Benedict about our diagnosis and medical management. He was not hired to educate him (or us) about GBS. But the lawyer in Mr. Benedict wanted his money's worth. He questioned his consultant like a star witness. It was all very cordial, even if the discussion at times sounded like a legal deposition. Dr. X, for his part, gave the information asked for.

Mr. B. "Of people who get this Guillain Barré, how many die from it?"

Dr. X. "Overall mortality is about 3%. That's in our experience and in other large series as well."

Mr. B. "What do the patients die of?"

Dr. X. "Three things, mainly. Heart disease, for one. This is usually associated with autonomic dysfunction, such as arrhythmia. Another cause of death is pulmonary embolus, which is when a blood clot breaks off from the legs and travels to the lungs. The clot comes from lying in bed so long. To some extent this can be prevented by giving small doses of heparin. I should add that her doctors have given this treatment all along." (At the mention of "her doctors" Mr. Benedict gave a slow and approving nod.)

"The third major cause of death in our patients is infection, such as pneumonia or septicemia. So far there seems to be no evidence for any of these problems in Mrs. Benedict."

Mr. B. "Is there any way to prevent the other two complications, the heart disease and infection?"

Dr. X. "Only by good care and catching the problems when they arise. One area of our research is the autonomic heart

problem. So far we haven't found a way to predict who will
develop it or why. That's why it's so important to watch GBS
patients closely, so you can treat the blood pressure crisis or
arrhythmia as soon as they occur. Mrs. Benedict had one such
crisis two days ago and it looks like she came out of it OK."

Mr. B. "But you agree with the plasmapheresis therapy?"

Dr. X. "Oh, absolutely. Apart from time, it's the only
effective treatment we can offer these patients."

Mr. B. "If this was your wife, would you do anything
different? Anything at all?"

Dr. X. "Mr. Benedict, if this was my wife I would not change
a thing. And if my wife happened to be in this hospital, with this
condition, I would not transfer her to New York. I would leave
her right where she is."

That is exactly what Mr. Benedict wanted to know.

* * *

That first week in MICU Naomi could only move her eyes,
eyelids, and some facial muscles. She managed a weak smile but
was unable to open her mouth wide or turn her head. Even so,
Mr. Benedict decided the children should see their mother. His
story about "infection" was wearing thin and the kids — a six-
year-old boy and ten-year-old girl — began to wonder out loud if
Mommy was dead.

I was ambivalent about the kids seeing their mother paralyzed.
They last saw her the morning of hospitalization. A visit when
she was still paralyzed could help or hurt her, and I wasn't sure
which. I suggested to Julian that he seek Naomi's opinion and he
agreed. To his question ('Naomi, do you want the kids to come
here?') she vigorously moved her eyes up an down. Yes!

Arrangements were made for the afternoon of March 14, her
seventh day of hospitalization. The night before the visit Julian
tried to prepare the children, by explaining that Mommy was too
weak to move and would not be able to talk, but that she loved
them very much, and that she would come home faster if they let
her know how much they loved and missed her.

About an hour before the appointed hour nurses tied Mrs.

Benedict's hair back in a bun and attached a pretty red ribbon. They also applied a small amount of makeup to her lips and cheeks. With the head of her bed raised to 45 degrees Naomi was sitting almost upright. Her head was buoyed by a pillow and turned to the left, so that she faced the side where her kids would stand. The tracheostomy tube and connecting hoses were covered discreetly with a bed sheet. From a distance Mrs. Benedict looked almost normal, like someone sitting in bed watching television.

Shortly after 4 p.m. Julian and the kids arrived. Both children were smartly dressed in school clothes. By pre-arrangement Julian took them straight to her room without any introductions to me or the staff. Worried about another autonomic surge, I discreetly stood in one corner of the room where she could not see me. Julian and the kids entered and walked to her bedside.

"Hi honey," said Julian. "I have Kevin and Cynthia with me."

Naomi managed a weak smile, an idiot-like grin the kids had never seen before. I saw it from across the room and shivered. Kevin and Cynthia just stood there, staring at their mother. For a few seconds — it seemed like a few minutes — no one said anything. I wondered: Did we make a mistake, letting them see her like this?

"Hi mom," said Cynthia, the ten-year-old. Thin and pretty, she was destined to be a beauty like her mother. "Hurry up and get well. We sure miss you. Daddy's taking good care of us."

"Mommy, this is for you," Kevin said, and he showed her an 8 x 11 inch picture he had drawn for the occasion. It displayed a red stick figure on a brown stick bed and big green block letters proclaiming GET WELL MOM SOON.

Mrs. Benedict wanted to smile and laugh and say what a wonderful picture it was, but all she could manage was the same feeble grin. Kevin didn't understand.

"Mommy, don't you like my picture? Mommy, why don't you hug me? I miss you Mommy!" He started to cry.

Cynthia nudged her brother and whispered sternly: "Kevin, Mommy can't hug you. She can't move right now."

The boy jumped away from Cynthia and tried to climb into his mother's bed. Julian pulled him back and he started to scream and cry louder. "MOMMY! MOMMY! MOMMY!"

Tears welled up in Naomi's eyes. Suddenly I felt awful. What must she feel? How unfair! Why had we let them come in? I wanted to leave and let Julian handle this visit in his own way but the cardiac monitor showed an accelerating heart rate. One hundred ten. One hundred twenty. One hundred sixty.

Although we needed to treat her quickly I spoke up without trying to sound excited or anxious. "Julian, I think we'll have to give her something. You better take them outside." He looked at me and I pointed to the cardiac monitor.

"Let's go kids," he said, and ushered them out.

*   *   *

The next two weeks were dismal for the Benedicts. Lack of any clinical improvement was wearing Julian down. One telephone conversation after a plasmapheresis treatment on March 20:

"Hi Larry, any change?" (By then we were on a first name basis).

"Not yet Julian. How are the kids?"

"Oh, they're fine. No permanent damage. They're just waiting for Mom to come home."

"I know. This is difficult for them. Well, tell them she will be home. And tell yourself that, too. It just takes time for the nerves to regenerate. If she remains stable she should improve."

Fortunately there were no more autonomic crises, no more emotional upheavals. Just the paralysis. Day after day of paralysis.

Then a change. Twenty days and six plasmapheresis treatments after coming to the hospital Mrs. Benedict began to move her *right index finger*. Regeneration!

"You're getting better," I told her. "You really are." We noted another big change: a broad, deep smile, far from the idiot grin displayed when her kids visited. I called Julian to relay the good news.

"How long will it take her to fully recover?" he asked.

"I don't know. Dr. McAllister says it could still take months, but at least nerve regeneration has started."

Without exercise — even the passive variety — paralyzed muscles develop disuse atrophy. Even after the nerve tissue regenerate the muscles can remain severely weak even. Since day one we had provided range of motion exercises to Naomi's paralyzed limbs. Despite the exercises (and tube feedings) there was some loss of muscle mass and her weight was down twenty pounds at the end of three weeks. She needed more exercise. From the orthopedics department we arranged to borrow a mechanical exerciser, a machine that continually moves the leg or arm to help maintain muscle tone. The machine is used mainly to exercise limbs after orthopedic surgery but we have also found it useful in some paralyzed patients.

Naomi had full sensation in her extremities so we alerted her to possible pain. "This contraption will keep your muscles fit," I explained. "If it causes you any pain or discomfort blink your eyes rapidly."

We secured her right leg to the exerciser. First the machine extended her leg. Then flexed it. Extended, flexed. Extended, flexed. A full range of motion every 12 seconds. Fortunately, she felt no pain.

Naomi continued to improve and by the end of March she could move her arms and head, but could not write or hold a glass. Also, her breathing muscles were still very weak. Normally, we can generate enough muscle strength to suck up a column of water to a height of about 100 centimeters (39 inches). People with respiratory failure from muscle weakness can suck up no than 20 centimeters (8 inches). The first time we tested her respiratory muscle strength, three days after the tracheostomy, Naomi managed only 10 centimeters of 'sucking' pressure. Now it was up to 18 centimeters. Still low but increasing!

"You continue to improve," I said, "but we have to go a few more days before you can get off the machine. You'll make it. As soon as you do we're going to throw a big party. If it's OK with you we'll keep it private. No one from the media will be invited." She smiled the equivalent of a hearty laugh.

We kept at it. Range of motion exercises. Tests of breathing strength. Tube feedings. Constant monitoring. She had settled into MICU and was beginning to feel almost "at home." She knew all the nurses and felt comfortable with her surroundings. The trauma of her kids' visit was ancient history.

To keep her mind occupied Julian brought in cassette selections from Books on Tape, which she listened to through an ear plug. In two weeks she went through Mark Twain's *Life On The Mississippi*, *The Cardinal of the Kremlin* by Tom Clancy and *The Bonfire of the Vanities* by Tom Wolfe.

* * *

On April 12 her inspiratory force was 24 centimeters of water. We disconnected the ventilator and gave her supplemental oxygen through the tracheostomy tube. Now, for the first time in over a month she was breathing entirely on her own. Since her inspiratory muscle strength was still 'borderline' I put her back on the ventilator after two hours.

"You did just great," I said, "but I don't want you to tire out. It's best if we do this a little bit each day. Tomorrow you'll go for four hours off the ventilator."

She moved her lips: "Where's my party?"

Naomi improved almost as rapidly as she had crashed. The next day her inspiratory force was 30 centimeters. I took her off the ventilator with the understanding that she would be re-connected after four hours.

For three hours and forty-five minutes there was no sign of fatigue or respiratory distress. Encouraged, I told the nurses to leave her off the machine indefinitely, with the idea that she might go the whole night unassisted.

Fifteen minutes later Naomi asked to see me. She had recently regained some use of her writing hand and was now communicating with paper and pencil. She wrote: BACK ON THE MACHINE?, meaning the ventilator.

"How do you feel?"

TIRED

I checked her respiratory rate, inspiratory force, cardiac rhythm, and blood pressure. They all pointed to one fact: physiologically, she didn't *need* the ventilator. Psychologically was another matter.

"Do you think you still need the breathing machine?" I asked.
YES

"Do you want to try and go without it a few more hours?"
NO

I have seen this response many times. Removing a patient from prolonged artificial ventilation often requires physiologic *and* psychologic adjustment. It makes sense. What has been critical life support is being discontinued; even though the patient no longer needs it, the "weaning" process takes time.

"OK," I said. "I think one more night. We'll put you back on the ventilator tonight. Tomorrow morning we'll disconnect it and let you go all day. If you do well during the day you'll be able to go all night without it. I promise." She liked the plan.

On April 14 she went all day without needing or asking for the ventilator. And all night. On April 15 we had our party.

Epilogue

Naomi Benedict continued to recover muscle strength. She began swallowing food on April 18 and regained movement in her legs by April 21. On that date we removed her tracheostomy tube. On April 25 she was transferred out of intensive care to the hospital's rehabilitation unit.

As expected she required extensive physical rehabilitation. On May 8, with the aid of a lightweight aluminum walker to keep balance, she took her first unassisted steps in two months. She went home from the hospital May 10.

Naomi continued muscle training exercises as an outpatient. Though progress was slow recovery was total. She started driving again in the middle of July and by September was back to a full schedule of meetings, parties, and charitable activities. She reports that Kevin and Cynthia are none the worse for her two month absence and that life is back to normal.

The only scar from her ordeal is physical and small, where the tracheostomy tube entered her neck. She usually covers it with a high collar blouse.

BIBLIOGRAPHY

In a collection of stories about intensive care, what should serve as bibliography? And is one even needed? The answer to the latter question is yes, for two reasons. *"Pickwickian" and Other Stories of Intensive Care* follows a long tradition of doctors and nurses writing about their patients. I would be remiss not to mention some of these other works, especially contemporary books still in print. The second reason is that several stories in this book raise important issues of medical ethics, issues that have been discussed in great detail elsewhere.

Hence this bibliography includes: 1) other first-person accounts that touch on intensive care, particularly those written for a general audience; 2) important articles and books that discuss ethical issues relating to intensive care. Although the articles are from medical journals, all can be understood by the lay reader.

Both listings are necessarily short and highly selective, and are meant to serve only as a guide.

FIRST-PERSON ACCOUNTS BY PHYSICIANS OR NURSES
(listed in alphabetical order by author)

Dan, Bruce B. and Young, Roxanne K. *A Piece of My Mind*. American Medical Association, 1988.
> A collection of short human-interest pieces by physicians and about patients, all of which appeared in the Journal of the American Medical Association during the 1980s.

Gino, Carol. *The Nurse's Story*. The Linden Press/Simon and Schuster, New York, 1982.
> A first-person account based on the author's 16 years in the profession.

(continued)

FIRST-PERSON ACCOUNTS (continued)

Hellerstein, David. *Battles of Life and Death.* Houghton Mifflin Co., Boston, 1986.
> Experiences of a sensitive and insightful doctor-in-training.

Heron, Echo. *Intensive Care. The Story of a Nurse.* Ballantine Books, New York, 1987.
> A first-person account by a nurse who has seen it all, in the emergency room and intensive care units.

Huttman, Barbara. *Code Blue. A Nurse's True-life Story.* William Morrow and Co., Inc., 1982.
> The first-person account of a middle-aged housewife who enters nursing school to learn what makes hospitals tick — and is told she has terminal cancer just before graduation. A very insightful and well-written book.

Klitzman, Robert. *A Year-Long Night. Tales of a Medical Internship.* Viking Penguin Inc., New York, 1989.
> An excellent first-person account of the internship year.

Kra, Siegfried, M.D. *The Three Legged Stallion and Other Tales from a Doctor's Notebook.* W.W. Norton Company, New York, 1989.
> Twelve fascinating medical stories by a cardiologist.

Kraegel, Janet and Kachoyeanos, Mary. *"Just a Nurse."* E. P. Dutton, New York, 1989.
> The authors, both registered nurses, use the interview technique to allow other nurses to tell their real-life experiences in nursing. Covers all areas of the hospital including intensive care.

Marion, Robert. *The Intern Blues.* William Morrow and Co., New York, 1989.
> A year in the mid-1980s spent caring for sick children.

Mullan, Fitzhugh. *Vital Signs. A Young Doctor's Struggle with Cancer.* Farrar Straus Giroux, New York, 1975.
One physician's account of his battle with almost-fatal cancer. Although written in the mid-1970s, anyone undergoing seemingly impersonal, high-tech care in the 1990s will appreciate this book.

Selzer, Richard. *Confessions of a Knife.* Simon and Schuster, New York, 1979.
Essays by a famous surgeon-author.

ARTICLES AND BOOKS ON MEDICAL ETHICS (listed in chronologic order)

Blackhall LJ. Must we always use CPR? New England Journal of Medicine 1987; vol. 317, pages 1281-85.

Macklin, Ruth. *Mortal Choices. Bioethics in Today's World.* Pantheon Books, New York, 1987.

Tomlinson T, Brody H. Ethics and communication in do-not-resuscitate orders. New England Journal of Medicine 1988; vol. 318, pages 91-5.

Ethical standards of medical practice. American College of Physicians Ethics Manual. Annals of Internal Medicine 1989; vol. 111, page 334.

Frankl D, Oye RK, Bellamy PE. Attitudes of hospitalized patients toward life support — a survey of 200 medical inpatients. American Journal of Medicine 1989; vol. 86, pages 645-48.

(continued)

ARTICLES AND BOOKS ON MEDICAL ETHICS (continued)

Murphy DJ, Murray AM, Robinson BE, Campion EW.
Outcomes of cardiopulmonary resuscitation in the elderly.
Annals of Internal Medicine 1989; vol. 111, pages 199-205.

Podrid PJ. Resuscitation in the elderly: A Blessing or a curse?
Editorial. Annals of Internal Medicine 1989; vol. 111:193-95.

Raffin TA, Shurkin JN, Sinkler W. *Intensive Care. Facing the Critical Choices*. W.H. Freeman and Company, New York, 1989.

Wanzer SH, et al. The physician's responsibility toward hopelessly ill patients. A second look. New England Journal of Medicine 1989; vol. 320, pages 844-49.

Wennberg, RN. *Terminal Choices. Euthanasia, Suicide, and the Right to Die*. Wm B. Eerdmans Publishing Co., Grand Rapids, MI, 1989.

Tomlinson T, Brody H. Futility and the ethics of resuscitation. Journal American Medical Association 1990; vol. 264, pages 1276-80.

Hackler, JC, Hiller FC. Family consent to orders not to resuscitate. Journal American Medical Association 1990; vol. 264, pages 1281-83.

Smedira NG, Evans BH, Grais LS, et al. Withholding and withdrawal of life support from the critically ill. New England Journal of Medicine 1990; vol. 322, pages 309-15.

Council on Ethical and Judicial Affairs, American Medical Association. Guidelines for the appropriate use of do-not-resuscitate orders. Journal American Medical Association 1991; vol. 265, pages 1868-71.

GLOSSARY

apnea - absence of breathing.

arterial - pertaining to the arteries, e.g. arterial blood.

arterial blood gas - refers to the pressure of oxygen and/or carbon dioxide in arterial blood; abbreviated ABG. An 'ABG' test routinely measures pressures of both gases, along with the level of blood acidity.

arterial line - a thin tube inserted into a patient's artery, usually the radial artery, for purposes of monitoring blood pressure or drawing frequent arterial blood gases. This technique is only used in intensive care units or in the operating room.

artery - blood vessel that carries oxygen-rich blood from the heart to the body's organs and tissues.

artificial ventilation - method of supplementing or taking over a patient's breathing with a machine (ventilator). The patient is connected to the ventilator via an endotracheal tube inserted through the mouth or nose.

artificial ventilator - see ventilator.

biopsy - removal of a piece of tissue from some part of the body for diagnosis.

blood gases - general term for carbon dioxide and oxygen in the blood; see arterial blood gas.

bronchitis - inflammation or infection of the airways (bronchi).

bronchodilator - a drug that relaxes airway smooth muscle and helps open up narrowed airways; useful in treating asthma.

bronchoscope - see bronchoscopy.

bronchoscopy - procedure whereby a thin, flexible tube (the bronchoscope) is inserted, via the mouth or nose, into the lungs; used to visualize the airways and diagnose many lung diseases. A biopsy can be done through the bronchoscope.

carbon dioxide - colorless, odorless gas, a byproduct of normal metabolism; abbreviated CO_2. Carbon dioxide is excreted by the lungs through the natural process of ventilation.

catheter - a thin, plastic tube that can be inserted into part of the body, such as a blood vessel or the bladder.

catheterization - general term for inserting a tube into a blood vessel. In cardiac catheterization a thin tube (catheter) is inserted through a vein or artery and into the chambers of the heart.

coronary - pertaining to blood vessels that serve the heart muscle; so-called because they encircle the heart like a corona.

coronary care unit - area of hospital for patients with acute heart disease, including suspected or diagnosed heart attack.

dialysis - process of cleansing the blood of toxins; in *hemo*dialysis, used to treat kidney failure, blood is removed through a vein, passed through a special filter that removes the toxins, then returned to the patient.

diuretic - a drug that promotes urine flow.

dopamine - an intravenous drug used to raise a patient's low blood pressure. See pressors.

dyspnea - shortness of breath.

embolism - condition when a blood clot moves from one part of the body to another; in pulmonary embolism the clot moves from some region of the body to the lungs.

emphysema - a chronic pulmonary disease, usually due to smoking, that leads to shortness of breath and blockage of airflow.

encephalitis - inflammation of the brain; see encephalopathy.

encephalopathy - a general term for confusion due to global brain disease. There are many possible causes including encephalitis and lack of oxygen (hypoxic encephalopathy).

endoscopy - general term for insertion of a flexible, diagnostic tube (endoscope) into a hollow organ; gastrointestinal endoscopy involves inserting an endoscope into the stomach or intestines.

endotracheal tube - a hollow plastic tube, approximately a foot long and a centimeter in diameter, inserted through the mouth or nose and into the trachea. It is used to facilitate artificial ventilation.

hematocrit - percentage of blood volume comprised of red blood cells (oxygen-carrying cells); normal range for hematocrit is

38-45% in women, 42-50% in men.

hemodialysis - see dialysis.

hyperthyroid - elevated level of thyroid hormone, the hormone that regulates metabolism.

hyperventilation - over-ventilation or over-breathing. Hyperventilation is accompanied by a reduced carbon dioxide level in the blood.

hypothyroid - low level of thyroid hormone.

hypoventilation - under-ventilation or under-breathing. Hypoventilation is always accompanied by an elevated carbon dioxide level in the blood.

hypoxemia - low oxygen level in the blood. Hypoxemia can manifest as either a low oxygen pressure (PO_2) or a low oxygen saturation; see PO_2.

intravenous - refers to route for medication or fluids given directly into a vein.

intubation - the placement of an endotracheal tube into the patient's airway, usually for purposes of providing artificial ventilation; see artificial ventilation.

meningitis - inflammation of the meninges, the thin membrane that covers the brain and spinal cord.

MICU - medical intensive care unit; area of the hospital for acutely ill adult patients, excluding those with surgical problems or primary cardiac disease.

mycoplasma - a bacteria-like organism that can cause pneumonia.

nitroprusside - an intravenous drug used to lower a very high blood pressure; is only administered in an intensive care unit.

pneumonia - infection of the lung tissues; can arise from many different types of micro-organisms, e.g. bacteria and viruses.

O_2 - Chemical symbol for oxygen.

oxygen - essential element of life; a colorless, odorless gas that comprises 21% of earth's atmosphere. Abbreviated O_2.

Pickwickian syndrome - term used to characterize a patient who is obese, falls asleep easily during the day and has an elevated level of blood carbon dioxide.

plasmapheresis - technique of separating out certain proteins from the plasma. Plasmapheresis is used to treat Guillain Barré syndrome and other illnesses.

PO₂ - Partial pressure of oxygen (O_2) in the blood. Any value for PO_2 above 60 is usually considered a safe level; lower than 60 indicates hypoxemia and potential danger for the patient.

pressors - intravenous drugs used to support or raise a low blood pressure. One commonly used pressor is dopamine.

psychosis - severe mental disturbance characterized by personality disintegration or some loss of contact with reality; schizophrenia is one form of psychosis.

respiration - general term for the process of bringing in oxygen from the atmosphere to the blood and excreting carbon dioxide from the blood to the atmosphere. Respiration is made possible by the process of breathing.

respirator - see ventilator.

respiratory failure - condition where the lungs have failed in their primary function of bringing adequate oxygen to the blood and of excreting carbon dioxide; in respiratory failure the level of blood oxygen is either reduced or the level of carbon dioxide is increased, or both.

sepsis - infection involving the blood stream.

tachycardia - fast heart rate, usually over 100 beats per minute.

trachea - medical name for 'windpipe,' the airway that connects the back of the throat to the lungs. The trachea is the largest airway and divides into two bronchi.

tracheostomy - a surgical procedure that places a hole in the trachea, through which is inserted a short (usually plastic) tube. Tracheostomy is almost always done on patients who need prolonged artificial ventilation.

tuberculosis - disease caused by a bacteria called *mycobacteria tuberculosis*; abbreviated TB. TB usually involves the lungs but may also appear in any part of the body.

vein - blood vessel that carries venous blood from the tissues back to the heart; venous blood is low in oxygen. See arterial.

venous - pertaining to the veins, e.g. venous blood.

ventilation - a general term for the physiologic process of delivering fresh air to the lungs. The term is sometimes used interchangeably with respiration.

ventilator - a machine capable of taking over a patient's breathing, also called a respirator. See artificial ventilation.

Index

ACE (angiotensin-converting-
enzyme) inhibitors, 204-5
AIDS (acquired immune deficiency syndrome), 40-44, 75,
86, 187-92, 194-98, 223
alcoholism, 6, 67-72, 138, 208
AMBU bag, 7, 22, 53, 168, 221
antibiotics, 30-32, 37, 39, 40, 42,
46, 75-76, 85, 88, 114-16, 165,
187, 195-97
anti-hypertensives, 204-6
ARC (aids-related complex),
187-89, 191, 193
ARDS (adult respiratory distress
syndrome), 73-89
artificial ventilation, 9, 12-13, 18,
24, 32, 36, 41, 57, 59, 75-76,
78, 83, 89, 103, 105, 107, 114-
16, 133, 139-41, 143, 167 195-
96, 208, 218, 233
asthma, 4-6, 17, 45-55, 109, 130,
155, 215
autopsy, 72

Bactrim, 86, 192
Banting and Best, 97, 98, 100,
101
blood gases, 10, 12, 20, 24, 49,
81, 84, 88, 115, 126, 128,
130-33, 136, 173, 195
breast cancer, 163, 166-67, 174
bronchi, 192
bronchitis, 49, 103, 105
bronchoscopy, 39, 192, 193

calcium channel blockers, 205

carbon dioxide, 19, 24, 52, 79,
81, 115, 116, 119, 121, 124,
128, 130, 138-39, 170
chest x-ray, 39, 48-49, 73-75, 77,
82, 84-85, 87-88, 142, 158,
164, 170, 172-73, 177, 185,
191, 193
chlorothiazide, 205
cigarettes, 49, 71, 103, 105,
107-9, 111, 113-15, 118 123,
164 (see also tobacco
addiction)
cocaine, 145-51
coma, 18-21, 24-25, 91, 99,
137-45, 147-48, 195-96, 208,
214
corticosteroids, 47-48, 83, 164
CPAP (continuous positive
airway pressure), 125
CPR (cardiopulmonary
resuscitation), 7-8, 50, 136,
150, 159
CVA (cerebrovascular accident),
3-4 (see also stroke)

diabetes, 87, 91-102, 123
diabetic coma, 91, 99
dialysis, 7, 23-24, 31, 37, 83, 208
(see also hemodialysis)
diet and dieting, 123-24, 126-27,
133, 136
dilantin, 22-23
diuretics, 205
DNR (do not resuscitate), 9-10,
34-35, 59, 62, 147, 193,
195-97